WHEN THE

Earth Moves

WHEN THE
Earth Moves

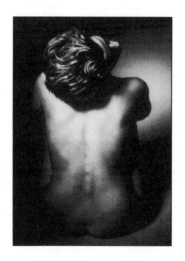

WOMEN AND ORGASM

MIKAYA HEART

CELESTIALARTS
Berkeley, California

CELESTIAL**ARTS**

P.O. Box 7123
Berkeley, California 94707
To order: order@tenspeed. com
Web site: www. tenspeed.com

Celestial Arts titles are distributed in Canada by Ten Speed Canada, in the United Kingdom and Europe by Airlift Books, in South Africa by Real Books, in Australia by Simon & Schuster Australia, in New Zealand by Tandem Press, and in Southeast Asia by Berkeley Books.

Cover and title page photo courtesy of Tony Stone Images
Cover design by Linda Davis at Star Type
Text design by Greene Design

Printed in Canada

Library Of Congress Cataloging in Publication Data:
Heart, Mikaya.
      When the earth moves : women and orgasm / Mikaya Heart
         p. cm.
      Includes bibliographical references (p.) and index.
      ISBN 0-89087-875-7 (pbk.)
      1. Sex instruction for women. 2. Female orgasm. 3. Women--
Sexual behavior. I. Title.
      HQ46.H416 1998
      613.9'6'082--dc21   98-38645
                                                                  CIP

1 2 3 4 5 6 7 / 05 04 03 02 01 99 98

I can lose myself completely in a powerful orgasm.
It's like being ripped out from inside.
It's like planets colliding.
Yes, the earth moves, but not before the Milky Way dissolves.

Acknowledgments

My heartfelt thanks go to all the following people:
Jesse Cougar, Caryn McClosky, Barbara Taylor, Joy Schulenburg, and Victoria Baker for their time, feedback, and support.

Barbara, Bonnie, Bluejay, Catrayl, Carolyn, Chris, Cora, D'Arcy, Deborah, Devorah, Diane, Donna, Doris, Jacq, Jana, Judy, Kay, Laurie, Linci, Lisa Sacks, Lisa Halse, Maggie, Maluma, Maria, Marya, Molly, Nancy, Nora, Nyna, Pat, Robin, Sage, Sari, Tine, Tui, Vika, and all the other wonderful women who spent time talking with me or filling in the questionnaire; also Bee, Dave, Rayner, and Wolfgang.

Thanks to my editor, Veronica Randall, and my agent, Nancy Ellis-Bell, for their enthusiasm and hard work, and to Veronica Randall and Linda Davis for a fantastic cover.

The following people had private conversations with me, which are quoted in part in the text of the book:
Lonnie Barbach, Ph.D, author of *For Yourself* and *For Each Other*, has worked with anorgasmic women for many years.

Joani Blank is a sex educator and therapist.

Jwala (415-995-4643) has been an international tantric teacher for twenty years. She is the author of *Sacred Sex: Ecstatic Techniques for Empowering Relationships*.

Dorrie Lane has a company called House O'Chicks, which makes sexually informative videos and the Wondrous Vulva Puppet.

Anna Marti is an intimacy coach, sex worker, and student of the erotic component of tantric disciplines. She works privately with individuals, couples, and groups throughout the country. Some of her quotes are from an interview with the Society for Human Sexuality (http://www.sexuality.org).

NightOwl is a pagan writer and sex activist. Her webpage is http://www.scn.org/ ~ nightowl. Some of her quotes are from an interview with the Society for Human Sexuality (http://www.sexuality.org/).

Annie Sprinkle spent eighteen years as a porn star, stripper, and prostitute. With the advent of the AIDS crisis, she became interested in sexual healing and erotic spirituality. She evolved into an internationally acclaimed avant-garde artist and feminist "pleasure activist". Some of her quotes are from her video *Sluts and Goddesses*.

Dr. Joan Spiegel is a sex therapist, psychologist, and homeopath.

David Steinberg is a columnist for *Spectator* magazine who has worked with men's groups for over twenty years. His two most recent books are *Erotic by Nature: A Celebration of Life, of Love, and of Our Wonderful Bodies* and *The Erotic Impulse: Honoring the Sensual Self*.

Deborah Sundahl is a sex activist who produces a video called *How To Female Ejaculate*. She is now producing another video on genital massage.

Patricia Huntington Taylor is author of *The Enchantment of Opposites: How to Create Great Relationships,* Traveling Artists Press.

The following people are quoted in the text of the book:
Carolyn Gage (carolyn.gage@maine.edu) is a lesbian author and playwright.

Catherine A. Liszt, is co-author of *The Ethical Slut: A Guide to Infinite Sexual Possibilities*. Greenery Press, 1997.

Alex Robboy, L.S.W., is a sex advisor on the Internet (alex@howtohavegoodsex.com).

Beverley Whipple, PhD, author and sexologist, who has done some wonderful work in the area of female sexuality, and Janet Lever, PhD, were both very helpful.

Table of Contents

Preface

I am fervently in support of opening ourselves up to unlimited passion. Human sexuality is both a great gift and a valuable tool that can enable us to get in touch with the wisdom and joy of our bodies, and help us to express our creativity. I believe that a healthy sex life makes for a healthy person, and I am unwilling to define what healthy means for anyone but myself. What I do in bed is based on what feels good to me, with my only limitation being that I never harm anyone else. I would like all of us to have the freedom to self-define, and I feel deeply grateful that I have been fortunate enough to reach a place in my life where I am able to enjoy unbridled sexual passion. It certainly wasn't always this way for me, and it still isn't this way for many women. It is my intention to illustrate the possibilities, and offer ideas to free up some of the glorious sexual energy that has been distorted and stifled by common misconceptions.

The women who are leading the way in the process of sexual reclamation are heterosexual, lesbian, and bisexual. But women who make love with other women have a vast body of firsthand information about women in particular, and have a unique outlook on female sexuality. Until recently, the lesbian perspective on sex was overlooked in this culture

because of homophobia, and because of the prevailing attitude that sex between two women is bound to be sweet,
nice, and "lesser than" sex with men. Standard definitions
have dictated that "real" sex must involve a penis. As a
lesbian myself, I'm well aware that this is far from the truth.
And this sorry misconception has prevented heterosexuals
(women *and* men) from taking advantage of a very useful
and fascinating perspective on sex. Therefore, while I have
included a high percentage of heterosexual input, much of
the information in this book is gleaned directly from lesbians. I feel enormously privileged to be in a position where
I can make "new" information and ideas available to the
general public. There has been a chasm of misunderstanding
and mistrust between heterosexuals and lesbians, and it will
be to everyone's benefit to bridge that chasm.

We live in a world of paradox, and nowhere is this paradox so apparent as in our attitudes to sex. On the one hand,
sex is glorified in the media; every time we turn on the television or look at a magazine cover we are presented with
messages about the power and allure of sex. And the sad
legacy of this is that many women die of anorexia every
year, trying to make themselves look attractive (read, skinny
and sexy). On the other hand, we are not supposed to have
sex with men outside marriage, or heaven forbid, with other
women. We are brought up to be demure, and women who
behave seductively are labeled whores or nymphomaniacs —
uncomplimentary epithets, to say the least. So in spite of its
glamorous veneer, many people still think of sex as
disgusting, and in some communities, as sinful. Although

men have been encouraged to experience a sex drive, their sensuality has been repressed. We have actually come to believe that "good" people are divorced from an awareness of their bodies, and "giving in" to our bodies' needs is considered a sign of weakness.

The mixed messages that bombard us are best summed up in the simple, though contradictory, lesson that many girls learn as they are growing up: *sex is dirty; save it for your husband.*

This society also trains us to invalidate our feelings. Throughout the book I frequently refer to the importance of paying attention to our feelings. I believe that it is virtually impossible to have good sex without having feelings. If you're going to be passionate, you have to allow yourself to feel passion!

We are now at a point in our cultural evolution when we are rediscovering the female, and finding a balance between the masculine and the feminine. Reversing negative messages, getting in touch with our feelings, acknowledging the healing power of our sexuality, and taking delight in our bodies' desires, are all part of establishing that balance.

As individuals, we must develop a sense of self-esteem that allows us to make our own choices, to take charge in a sexual setting, and find our own ways of getting our needs fulfilled, outside and beyond anyone else's moral judgments of what is right or wrong, good or bad, normal or abnormal . Many women are still afraid of asserting themselves sexually: they've been taught to put their own needs aside, make sure their lover has a good time, and pretend everything is fine.

For women there's a tremendous temptation to pretend you're having a better time than you're having, because women warm up so slow and men warm up so fast. There's an enormous temptation to hope your body will catch up if the sex goes on long enough, which is self-defeating because if you have sex before you're really hot it just doesn't feel that great. — NightOwl

Unfortunately, we live in a society where not all women are able to assert themselves. In the United States, a woman is battered every nine seconds, over four million women are battered annually, and four women are murdered daily as a result of domestic violence. (Casa Myrna Vazquez, Inc., http://www.tofias.com/skate.htm, 1998). The ideas and information in this book are not geared for women stuck in abusive situations. This information is for those women who are ready, willing, and able to claim their power. To these women I want to say: it's time to take responsibility for your own fulfillment.

A major part of such responsibility involves doing away with the taboos against talking about what we like and don't like when we're being sexual. When you ask a friend to come over and take care of your house while you're away, surely you don't expect her automatically to know where everything is? And yet, the first time you go to bed with someone, do you discuss what parts of your body you like to have touched, and how? Do you even try to explain what turns you on? Do you say what you like and don't like? Well, if not, how can you expect someone to know your preferences, any more than you can expect that person to know where everything is in your house?

4

I make a practice of telling any new lover, before we start being sexual, that I don't come very easily and I would rather she didn't try to make me come; if I want to come, and think that I will be able to, I will direct her. I also tell her what kind of stimulation I like or don't like, and I ask her what she likes. I've had some strange reactions ("Oh, you're so romantic!"), but I really don't care; I hate working in the dark, literally *and* figuratively. A lot of women have the idea that maintaining a romantic mood requires keeping any discussion of sex to the level of innuendo, and avoiding graphic detail. They are wrong.

I also made a rule with myself some years ago that I would never try to make someone come. As soon as that dynamic is set up, it changes what should be a delightful act of making love into a performance-oriented chore, something that is being done only with a goal in mind, rather than for the pure enjoyment of it. Obviously I want to give my partner pleasure. But I never want her to think that I won't be satisfied unless she has an orgasm. I know from personal experience that as soon as I begin to think that my partner is invested in me having an orgasm, or *needs* for me to come to give her a sense of her own fulfillment, then I cannot do it. I certainly don't want to exert the same pressure on my partner. I don't want orgasm to be something that is imbued with a sense of achievement, or lack thereof.

Many people believe that women *should* have orgasms, that there is something wrong with a woman if she doesn't. I don't believe this, any more than I think all women *should* be thin, or all women *should* drink herbal tea, or all women *should* learn to paint. I think that a woman who wants to have an orgasm will be able to do so in her own good time, when her body is ready for it. We need to stop defining sex as a merely physical function, and begin to acknowledge its emotional and spiritual depth. The pressure on a woman to have orgasms, and the opinion that if she doesn't there must be something wrong with her, can be deeply damaging, whether such notions come from "experts" or from her lover. Many women have good sex without having a conscious experience of something that can be labeled orgasm. The trouble is that if we're told we "ought" to be experiencing something we're not, then we're likely to feel inadequate. And we get trapped in a scarcity mentality.

Having orgasms, or not, is a personal thing. It varies as much as any other aspect of sexuality. Some women ejaculate, some don't. Some women enjoy penetration; some don't. Some women have huge orgasms; some have little ones. Some women have multiple orgasms; some women have one. Some women just aren't particularly sexual, and others are. If a woman really wants to learn to have an orgasm, she may well be able to do so. But it's sort of like learning to ride a bicycle: it's an unconscious trick of the mind in combination with the body that makes her suddenly able to balance, where she couldn't do so before. Having sexual feelings is all about experiencing flows of energy: blocking them or allowing them to flow. There are usually very good reasons why a woman will block a certain flow of energy at a particular time, even if those reasons (or the fact that she is blocking anything at all) are deeply buried in her unconscious. Releasing our passion, managing sexual and creative energy, is not usually something that can happen on a conscious level. It is related to the healing of the whole individual. What's important for all women is to go with what our bodies want. It may be that women who don't come or don't come easily, are not psychologically ready to experience what the orgasm will do to them: that intense, shocking alignment of body and soul that can occur with a strong orgasm.

From my own experience of talking to and making love with many different women, and from listening to the experiences of others, both heterosexual and lesbian, I believe there is a vast complexity of possibility in women's orgasm. There are many different kinds, varying from whole body orgasm to clitoral or vaginal, from mental orgasm to intensely emotional ones. Women can come in vastly different ways: some women need intense clitoral stimulation, and others can come from making love to someone else, never having their own genitals touched. It all seems to have to do with the way women experience the world, and the place of their own bodies within it. One woman might get enormous enjoyment out of wearing the color pink; another might think it's revolting. Some women get great pleasure from sucking a man's penis; other women think that's revolting. Some women might really enjoy the sensation of a wild carnival ride, but others might find it utterly terrifying. One woman may love to feel her body shaken by an intense orgasm, while another woman might find the onset of the orgasm to be so upsetting that she automatically stops it.

Social mores impose judgments on many of these things
— for instance, a young girl is more likely to get adult
approval for wearing a dress than for wearing overalls. We
put our own judgments on all of the above — for instance, I
feel like a wimp when I get carsick. Religious and political
thinkers all have their judgments: a radical lesbian feminist
might think it's just as wrong to suck on a man's penis as a
fundamentalist Christian would, making them unusual allies
indeed! But none of these judgments have any real value or
use in the world except to make the people who do like
those things feel defensive or bad about themselves.

What is orgasm? The truth is, I am not really interested in
producing a definition that applies universally. I think that
such a definition could never encompass the enormous variety of what women call orgasm. As you will discover as you
read further, there are women who can come as they walk
across a room, and there are women who don't come at all.
There are women who started having orgasms at the age of
four and there are women who started having them at the
age of sixty-four. The experience of orgasm is a highly
individual one, and the spectrum of experience is huge. For
some women, orgasm is an integral part of their sexuality,
and they expect to have dozens every time they make love;
other women are content *not* having orgasms in a definable
way, or would be content, if they weren't made to feel abnormal or freakish.

I am not interested in formulating complex theories of
sexuality. Defining what's what is always limiting. A
definition is merely a container, and it's all too tempting to

try to shove everything you think ought to belong there into it, whether it really fits or not. On the contrary, I am interested in broadening the scope of our thinking, and encouraging all of us to communicate openly and without shame about our sexuality. Freeing up our desires can bring us to a place of ecstatic celebration that is much more than physical. Getting over our fear of speaking openly about sex can be a cause for group celebration rather than one that is hidden away from our friends and confined to the bedroom. At the present time, sex is something that separates us from our communities. I am not suggesting we all start having group sex. And I am certainly not condoning sexual abuse of any kind. I am suggesting that, by talking openly about our sexuality, we can use it as a tool to bring us into community. I am suggesting that we talk about it in a real way — not just joking and laughing, not boasting, but saying what is real for us about sexual play: what works and what doesn't, what we fear as well as what we desire. I believe there is a very powerful potential for good in our sexuality.

I believe that if we were more open about sex, sexual abuse could become a rare occurrence. It is precisely the taboos around sex that make it possible for people to get away with molestation, shielded by a conspiracy of silence. Moreover, the prevailing stigma of shame forces some people to repress any desires that might be considered unacceptable. And repressed desires tend to grow. It is possible that a more enlightened and compassionate society could help disturbed people to find harmless outlets, and it's certainly possible to provide them with places to go for help: places where they would be prevented from harming others, but where they would not immediately be ostracized and condemned. The atmosphere of secrecy and denial surrounding sex promotes abuse, not only because it makes it easy for abusers to hide what they're doing, but also because it makes it hard for them to acknowledge that they need to find help. Encouraging people to talk about feelings and desires that are unacceptable does *not* mean we are condoning them. It means we are acknowledging that none of us is born perfect, and we are willing to work together to find ways of coexisting that don't damage other people.

We need to learn to validate and vocalize our sexual preferences, and I don't just mean who we go to bed with, whether it's someone of our own gender or the opposite gender: I mean what we do when we're in bed with that person, the feelings we have, the experience of loving that person; I mean the experience of loving ourselves and our bodies, what kinds of things are pleasurable for us. And what kinds of things *don't* feel good, what kinds of things would we prefer *not* to do.

I interviewed twenty-six women and three men in detail about their sex lives. You will find some of them referred to throughout the book. In addition, the questionnaire on page 336 was posted on the internet and circulated by hand prior to the publication of this book. Its purpose was to encourage women to think about their sexuality, and then put their thoughts down on paper for me to pass on to you, the reader. It is my hope that they shared it with their lovers and friends as well. The italicized quotes appearing throughout the book are from the questionnaire or from the interviews, and they are credited where the individual requested it. (See acknowledgments.) The questionnaire was never intended to provide statistics, since I did not have the resources to access a random sample of the population.

In 1994, the National Health and Social Life Survey (NHSLS) questioned over three thousand randomly selected Americans and came up with some statistics that are probably about as valid as any we are going to get on sexual behavior. I have quoted some of these statistics, and also some from a survey that was done worldwide by Durex, the condom manufacturer. None of these statistics are to be taken as gospel, for two reasons. Firstly, a statistic is only as good as its interpretation: if a higher percentage of well-educated women report performing oral sex, does this mean that you are more likely to engage in oral sex because you have a good education? Or, if you are the kind of person who likes oral sex, are you also likely to be someone who gets a good education? These are only two of a number of possible interpretations. And, of course, just because a number of well-educated women said they enjoyed oral sex does not mean all well-educated women like it!

Secondly, reality varies vastly from individual to individual; some people are very invested in maintaining their perceived reality, while others are very willing to question it. Thus, a woman with a traditional or conservative upbringing is more likely to say that she is satisfied because she is living according to society's code of approval, and therefore believes she ought to be satisfied, since society informs her that she ought to be satisfied. Her security may depend on her *not* questioning her life. (What would she do if she decided she wasn't satisfied? It may be unthinkable to her that she could be doing anything else with her life.) On the other hand, someone who has broken with traditional values is someone who has questioned what satisfaction is; she's probably someone who is not easily satisfied, and yet might be living what would appear, to some of us, to be a much richer existence than someone who has never questioned society's dictates. Her concept of satisfaction probably has wider parameters and is less easily reached.

In other words, a survey isn't always reliable when it concerns highly charged subjects that are steeped in moral judgment.

In some societies sex is regarded as a sacred act. In this society we have come to regard it as an act of profanity. Yet sex can be profoundly spiritual. Most women experience it as much more than a physical experience, and for many of us it can be deeply transformative and healing, bringing us to the realization that we are much more than physical bodies, confined by the limits of flesh and blood. We can choose to develop this kind of awareness by conscious sexual practice. As the sexual energy courses through our bodies, it opens channels to other levels of being. No matter what our sexual orientation may be, we can use sex as the doorway to a profound personal and spiritual awakening.

The paths that we take in our lifetimes are many and varied, no one exactly the same as another. When we follow them without preconceptions about where we ought to be going, they often take us to unexpected places. As someone who grew up with particularly unpleasant associations around sex, I never thought I might one day write a book on orgasm, yet this is where my path has led me.

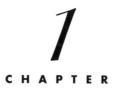

CHAPTER

Personal Experience

I need to be allowed to be sexual, to be encouraged to be sexual, to experience myself as a sexual being. When I'm in that place my energy is boundless and beautiful, and I am free, happy, and healthy.

I was born in 1952 in rural Scotland. A friend of the family molested me when I was a youngster; the trauma left me believing that sex was evil and dangerous. I grew up hating my body and convinced that nothing relating to sex should ever be talked about. I was also taught that, as a female, I did not have the right to say no, and did not have control over my own body. I understood that my needs were always secondary to those of men. So, by the age of fourteen, I was allowing my body to be used by various fumbling teenage boys, who were intent on proving their virility. My mind vacated my body for their use and I kept my gathering rage under wraps. I certainly never investigated my genital area. Why would I, when I had only experienced sex as intrusive and unpleasant?

It may be difficult to understand why I wasn't able to assert my right to say no. I was brought up in a social setting where great importance was placed on appearance. As long as everything appeared to be okay, it didn't matter what was actually going on. What mattered was that no one got upset in public. I learned to make light of any and all problems. The more upsetting something was, the more important it was to joke about it or ignore it. And that is how the subject of sexuality is generally treated. If it is treated seriously, it's usually only in an academic fashion. When I was growing up, there was no opportunity for me to express my distress about sex. This is still true for many children, teenagers, and adults today.

By observing the people around me, I concluded very early on in life that women were powerless and inferior to men. So I decided that I would grow up to be a man. I was appalled when I began to develop breasts. But my fate was irrevocable — I was going to be a woman. I might go to university, I might even have some kind of a career, but the fact that I was born without a penis meant that I should be married with children by the time I was thirty. I would be responsible for keeping the house clean and looking after the children and cooking for my husband and his friends. I would be dependent on my husband, whoever he might be, for money. My primary job would be catering to him.

Although I knew that everyone around me saw this as my destiny, I could never quite imagine it. I coveted the idea of independence, and couldn't imagine that I would ever willingly give it up once it was within my grasp. In the meantime, I made the best of my miserable circumstances. Having accepted that my place in the world was to be a woman, I utilized the only source of power I could — my ability to seduce men. I caved in to the pressure to give up my tomboy ways, learned to wear dresses, and made myself as sexy as I could. I flirted with boys at every opportunity until they succumbed to my charms, and then I dropped them. No, I didn't just drop them — I trampled them in the mud.

The disadvantage of this game was that I had to have sex with them, and that was never pleasant. I didn't see that I had a choice. I actually "lost my virginity" when I was very drunk at the age of seventeen. It's a sordid, all too common story and I won't go into it. But by the time I was eighteen, a strange thing happened — I started to enjoy sex. I still had no idea that such a thing as a clitoris existed. I was twenty-one before I realized that women were supposed to have something called an orgasm. I certainly never dreamed of talking about sex — that would have been far too exposing. However, in spite of all my negative conditioning, my body, of its own volition, occasionally responded eagerly during intercourse.

I wonder how different things would have been if I had been able to ask for what I wanted, or if any of the boys or men I went to bed with had had any idea how to give pleasure to a woman. I hope that this book may help teenagers to make more positive choices around sex, and to avoid the destructive power games of seduction that were the norm when I was a teenager.

Time passed. I stopped playing seduction games as I fell in with a different crowd of people. I became a hippie and dropped out of the environment that would have molded me into somebody's wife. I stopped wearing dresses altogether

— then and there I abandoned that persona completely (although it was some years before I came out as a lesbian). Slowly, I began to learn that I had a right to say no, although like most women, I only exercised that right when I was really sure I meant it. Since I did not regard ambivalence as adequate grounds for refusal, I still frequently acquiesced when I wasn't really sure. My priority was always to please my lover when we were in bed. I rarely thought seriously about what I wanted, and I tried to avoid any feelings that might be considered inappropriate. This is the coping mode of many women in many cultures. It doesn't make for satisfying, quality relationships.

When I was twenty-four, two of my close female friends persuaded me that in order to have an orgasm (which I'd finally decided I had not had, and they assured me I ought to be having), I should learn to masturbate. I was beginning to feel a little better about my body, so I made myself practice touching my genitals. I didn't enjoy it a whole lot, but I dutifully lay in bed at night and manipulated that sensitive little nub of flesh that I figured must be my clitoris.

All Work and No Play

At first it was too much work, and I stopped as soon as I got to the edge of something that felt uncomfortable. I didn't think that uncomfortable sensation could lead to an orgasm, because orgasms were supposed to feel "good." But more conversations with my friends informed me that I should push past the point of discomfort. I returned to work. One night, when the tension in my body built to that now familiar place, I gritted my teeth and kept going. The sensation became unbearably intense. I stopped and let my breathing return almost to normal. Then I continued. Following my body's demands, I stretched out my legs until the muscles in my calves were aching. I stopped and tried to relax, and forced myself to carry on. My shoulders, my neck, and my belly became as tight as iron and I felt as though I was going to explode — and it wasn't going to feel good. But something else was happening; an urgent feeling had built specifically in my pelvic area, and this feeling seemed to have a life of its own. I had a sense that something astonishing, something much more powerful than I was carrying me like a wave, and then it flung me down on the shore. I lay there panting and exhausted, feeling bruised and shaky. My calves hurt like hell, my clitoral area felt like it had been burnt, I was trembling all over, and I wanted to cry. I curled up and held myself, comforting myself with the thought that I never had to do this again. Powerful aftershocks racked my body for several minutes.

Could my first orgasm have been a better experience? If I had been brought up in a sex-positive environment, I believe my whole history, sexual and otherwise, would have been much better.

As you can imagine, I wasn't too happy about my venture into the realm of orgasm. My friends persuaded me that it would improve with practice. However, something else happened right around this time, something that changed my life completely: without any premonition that I would do so, I fell in love with a woman. Sex with her was completely different from anything I had ever experienced before. For the first time in my life I understood why the sex act was called "making love." It was my first encounter with the concept of love.

We had a passionate affair, she left me, and I set out to find other women. I embraced the label "lesbian." For a while I was in bliss: deeply grateful for my woman-ness, and for the complete acceptance of other lesbians. I very quickly left behind all my body hatred. I loved other women's bodies, and as a result I loved my own. Those feelings have stayed with me to this day. Ever since I became aware of my attraction to women, I have been very thankful that I was born female.

Sex with women was a completely different experience than it was with men. I became more aroused and felt emotionally connected in a way I never had before. But it wasn't exactly a bed of roses, or at least it had plenty of thorny areas. Had I remained with men, I would probably not have bothered much with orgasms. But my female partners wanted me to come and they noticed if I didn't. I tried diligently, both because I wanted to make them happy, and because I wanted to be a functional and healthy person. And I now believed that functional and healthy women had orgasms.

Some of the time I did manage to come, but it was a couple of years before orgasms became relaxing or fulfilling. Mostly they were more agonizing hard work than anything else. I thought I was taking far too much time coming, and I worried that my lover would get bored, or would be alarmed (as I was) by the way my legs would jerk for several minutes, even as long as half an hour, after I'd come. Gradually I began to learn to manage my sexual energy, and I got to the point where I could actually achieve a fairly complete release, so that I was not left with an uncomfortable sense of inner vibration. It helped when I realized that I need to come several times in one session.

I still didn't talk about sex very much, and still didn't feel able to ask for what I wanted. I rarely thought about it: in fact, I was careful not to, but if I had articulated what was going on for me at this time, I would have had to say that I felt it was not okay for me to be in touch with what I really wanted. I lived in a lesbian feminist community where there was great pressure to be politically correct in thought, word, and deed. This even extended to what you did in bed, and one of the things you were not supposed to want was penetration. I did enjoy oral sex, but the truth was I also desired penetration. I didn't want to admit that at the time, even to myself.

More than that, I felt that I could not tell my lover how to make love to me for fear of offending her. I somehow thought that I should like what she liked to do to me. I felt too inadequate and insecure to say anything if I didn't. Like many women, I occasionally faked orgasm to avoid dealing with the ramifications of why it wasn't happening for me. Faking was not an active lie, it only involved omitting to mention that I hadn't come. Instead, I would act like I wanted more and wanted it harder, which I often did.

Into the West

Time passed, and strict views on sexual behavior began to soften. Meanwhile I moved to northern California. This provided me with opportunities I had not had in Britain. Firstly, it was much easier for me to heal from the wounds left over from my childhood. I worked on my old emotional pain with some excellent therapists, and after a few years I succeeded in reversing many of my ingrained childhood beliefs about sex and about being a woman. I began to feel that it was perfectly fine for me to be who I was and want what I wanted.

Secondly, moving to California provided more opportunities to meet and be lovers with women who were already free in their sexuality. Encouraged by my lovers, I began to play around with a variety of sexual practices, including penetration, and I found that it added a whole new dimension to sex. While I still need (and enjoy) clitoral stimulation in order to have what I recognize as an orgasm, I have peaks of enjoyment during penetration that are a different kind of climax. And I like to experience penetration at the same time as I am having my clitoris stimulated, so that I can come with something inside me, which makes my orgasms much fuller.

I began to talk with my lovers about the nuts and bolts of being sexual: the actual nitty-gritty of tongues and hands and clits and vaginas. I even began to venture into the land of sex toys. The more women I made love with, and the more open those women were willing to be with me, the more amazed and delighted I became at the diversity of our sexual responses. My sex life blossomed.

Of course I had heard about Freud's theories on female orgasm, and I had long ago dismissed the concept of a vaginal orgasm as ridiculous, since all the women I had been with, up to that point, liked to have clitoral stimulation along with penetration, or without any penetration at all. For years I had firmly believed that all orgasms were clitorally based. Then I began to ask other women what they thought, and found that a number of them related to the concept of a vaginal orgasm. When I finally found Judy, who has very clearly separate vaginal and clitoral orgasms, all my questions and speculations began to coalesce into the idea of writing a book.

I cannot stress too strongly how deeply healing it has been for me just to talk about sex. Speaking openly and honestly about my desires and listening to other women speak openly and honestly about theirs has released me from the veil of shame that shrouded the subject of sex when I was growing up. It has also been, and continues to be, incredibly informative. The learning process is ongoing. Our bodies are capable of the most extraordinary things, particularly when they are in a state of sexual arousal. And what limits our sexuality are the concepts we cling to of what we think is *meant* to happen.

A New Vocabulary for Sex

Sex is like life. Our concepts of what sex is are shaped by our expectations; our expectations are shaped by our culture and our culture is shaped by, and shapes, our language. At the present moment we have a very limited language to express what sex is and what our sexual experiences are. In order to expand our view of sex, which is essential for most people if they are going to experience true fulfillment, we need to alter and expand our language. This can only happen if people are willing to communicate openly about sex.

Although I know that not everyone will agree with me on a clear-cut definition of what sex is, I think most people would agree that, at least some of the time, sex is about love. I have heard women say that they are tired of fucking, and they want to be making love. I believe what they mean is that they want their sexual play to involve a heart-and-soul connection, or that they want to settle down with one partner. These two situations are by no means always the same!

Either way, they are using the word "fucking" in a derogatory sense, to mean sex that isn't really loving. I don't personally use it that way, I use it to mean the act of penetration. Until a few years ago, the word had the same derogatory connotations for me as it does for most people: it indicated something vulgar, coarse, a little bit disgusting. Why did it change for me? I think because I gradually began to need a functional word that described a physical act (penetration) that was pleasurable and at the same time denoted an instinctively animal passion.

I am careful where I use the word fucking because of the derogatory spin it carries for most people. I try to use it only in situations where it is clear that I mean it positively. Sadly, sex can be sordid, and often is. But for me, my sexual play, whether it involves fucking or not, is about "making" love. I make lots of love when I'm being sexual. I often feel filled up with love; I feel surrounded by love; I feel open and vulnerable, and powerful in my vulnerability.

When you truly let your sexual energy flow freely throughout your entire being, you'll feel as though you're making love every moment of every day with everything and everyone — *even during a root canal.* — Annie Sprinkle

For the sake of clarity, I often use the terms **doer** and **receiver**. The receiver is the one who is having something done to her, and might appear to be the more passive partner; the doer is the one who is doing, and might appear to be the more active partner. (Obviously there are times when this division is meaningless.)

The other term I frequently use is **sexual play**. It is vital that we begin to define sex as a playful exchange, so that the games we engage in and the roles we adopt are openly acknowledged and discussed between willing participants. I do not use the term "foreplay," since it denotes a goal, a beginning and an end, and I've never related to it. While there are (possibly) beginnings and ends to particular acts during particular sexual encounters, sexual undercurrents are going on all the time, between all kinds of people. Whether or not we choose to bring these undercurrents to the surface, and act on them, should *always* be the result of consensual agreement between adults.

Traditional sexual interchanges all too often involve one person initiating an act that the other person feels ambivalent about, due to her past experience, or the likelihood that she won't get her needs met, or both. **Consensuality** and

negotiation are extremely important concepts that are sadly lacking in this kind of exchange. Good sex must always be fully consensual, which means that both partners consciously agree to it, rather than doing things a certain way by default. Women rarely have a clear concept of their right to define what happens to them in their lives generally. Until we assert our right to self-definition in all our interchanges, we cannot be fully present. And even then, it may take a long time to make meaningful changes in the sexual arena.

The Best Medicine

One of the main problems we have with sex is a lack of playfulness. Instead of a natural act that has a flow of its own and arises out of a healthy desire, it often becomes stilted and laden with "issues"; it becomes something that we are afraid of or something that we desperately want, and either way we are terrified of failing at it. We try to make it flawless, perfect, romantic, and our need to have it this way only leads to tension and awkwardness.

The times I remember best are the times when there was laughter as well as passion.

The best antidote to an overdose of seriousness is laughter; I'm not talking about the inane "dirty" jokes that reinforce tiresome and damaging stereotypes, but loving laughter that stems from a down-to-earth feeling of joy. Whether it's a giggle or a good deep belly laugh, it's wonderful when lovers can roll around together in hilarity. The things that we get so anxious about, be they lack of orgasm, lack of erection, or anything else, are exactly the things that don't have to matter at all, and we need to learn to be flippant about them. If a man could look down at his limp penis and say, "Uh-oh, looks like it's not coming out to play today," or a woman, instead of faking it, could say, "I can see this orgasm out of the corner of my eye, but I think it's running the other way," then we'd be able to relax and have a good time, instead of fixating on what's *not* happening.

Being goofy and playful takes me a lot further. Laughing breaks down a certain barrier that makes it possible to open up more sexually.

Laughter can also be part and parcel of an orgasm.

Once we were making love in a place where we had to be really quiet, and when my lover came she was desperately trying to stifle her moans, but they kept breaking through as loud snorts, a mixture of laughter and sexual pleasure. We both laughed helplessly for several minutes, and the ripples of suppressed laughter shook my body just like an orgasm.

These days, sex is laden with fear of disease, and it may be difficult to be spontaneous. All the more reason to be able to laugh, as you drop the condom on the floor, or it splits as you're putting it on, or you roll off the edge of the bed as you're reaching for it.

When the telephone by the bed rang, I reflexively picked it up. It was a repairman telling me what was wrong with my computer and how difficult it would be to fix. And here I am, on my hands and knees, getting it really hard and really well doggie-style with this huge hard dick, on the verge of coming, and more or less shouting into the phone, "Oh yeah, whatever it takes, just do it. Do it. Do it! DO IT!!!" And, the nice thing was, they both listened to me and did it. . .

I would like the reader to understand that most of the women I have interviewed are unusual; they are the ones who have been willing (and often eager!) to talk about what sex is for them. Their experiences represent some of the possibilities within the range of female sexuality.

Because I don't want to leave the reader with the idea that we are all having sex as good as those of us who are happy to talk about it, I have made an effort to include some women who are not satisfied with their sex lives. I am extremely grateful to the women who are not confident in their sexuality, for being willing to talk to me; I know it wasn't easy for them and I feel their input is extremely important in revealing the truth — that many women today have not yet experienced sexual fulfillment.

Safer Sex

In this day and age it would be irresponsible to write a book on sex without including some information on the risk of disease. I prefer the phrase saf*er* sex to *safe* sex, since we do not know enough about modes of transmission to be certain of being absolutely safe, and the only completely safe course of action is no action, that is, abstinence. Safer sex is a more viable option for many of us.

Some diseases, such as herpes and chlamydia, are spread primarily by sexual contact, and others, such as hepatitis and

HIV, the virus that causes AIDS, can be spread by a variety of methods, including sexual contact. One of the most common modes of transmission for AIDS is shared needles among intravenous drug users. There are some high-risk professions, also, including healthcare workers who routinely come into contact with blood products.

While it is impossible to lead a life in which you will never be exposed to any kind of disease, it is also true that a little care goes a long way. I believe it is unethical to omit some basic precautions. It is a little like crossing the road: if you run out into the middle of a busy freeway (equivalent to having unprotected sex with everyone you meet) and expect to remain uninjured, you're living in a fool's paradise. But if you always wait until you can see no moving vehicles in either direction before you step out (equivalent to never having sex at all), then you will spend a lot of your life standing anxiously on the sidewalk. You may stay alive, as long as some crazy driver doesn't mount the sidewalk to mow you down.

You may get tired of hearing this, but the most important factor is honest and open communication with your partner. Discuss your sexual and health history with *all* potential partners. Make an agreement about what kind of precautions you are going to take, and *stick to them*. It's vital to be able to trust your long-term or short-term partners not to violate your agreements. There is a behavior continuum from ultrasafe: "If it's wet and it's not yours, then don't touch it;" to safer (better than no precautions at all): using condoms for vaginal or anal intercourse but not for fellatio, for instance. You may decide to use no barriers with a primary partner, but to be very careful to avoid any exchange of body fluids with all other partners.

You want your partner to be honest with you, so be honest with your partner. But you should not base a decision not to do safe sex on what your partner tells you; people who have diseases tend to be stigmatized and this makes it hard for them to tell the truth. Moreover, illegal drug use and unsanctioned sex (sex outside marriage or sex with a prostitute, for instance) are things that even usually trustworthy people may lie about.

If you have sex with multiple partners, you and your partners should get tested regularly for HIV. Testing is available that is totally anonymous, absolutely free and no longer involves having blood taken, since there is now an accurate saliva test. However, if you do contract the virus, it may take up to six months to show up in your blood. So be aware that even if you have a negative test result, you could be carrying the virus if you have indulged in risky practices within the previous six months.

If you are in a monogamous relationship, and have been so for at least six months, and you have recently had a negative AIDS test, don't work in a high risk profession, and don't share needles, then your only concern is that you are not carrying any other disease, such as hepatitis, chlamydia, genital warts, syphylis, gonorrhea, or herpes.

I recommend the following as basic safety precautions:

1 Get regular checkups. Chlamydia can cause sterility in women, yet its symptoms are often minimal or non-existent. A herpes flare-up will go away of its own accord, but

it means you are a herpes carrier, and you need to know that so that you don't pass it on to others. If you have any kind of sores on your labia, or any sign of a discharge, go to a doctor.

2 Use condoms. Don't just think about them — use them. Use them regularly, as a habit. Use them on dildoes, use them on penises. Use them for vaginal intercourse, use them for anal intercourse, use them for oral sex. If your partner objects, discuss alternatives. These might be no intercourse of any kind or using a vaginal condom (the Reality female condom is available from any sex store, but it needs a little practice to use properly). There are many kinds of condoms, and some are much more comfortable and allow more sensitivity than others. Try different kinds. To increase sensation, try applying a little lube before you put the condom on.

Condoms occasionally break (usually because they are not put on correctly). Learn how to put them on properly. If you want extra safety, try using two together, but put a little lube in between them so they don't stick to each other, which would make them more likely to break.

3 Use latex gloves (or some other kind if you are allergic to latex). They are inexpensive and easy to use. If your hands are very clean and free of cuts or abrasions, and you're not using them for heavy penetration, gloves are not absolutely essential. But have a box by your bed for the times when your hands have cuts on them or you're doing anal penetration, or fisting (vaginal or anal).

4 If you are performing cunnilingus or anilingus, use dental dams, female condoms, a glove cut open (with your tongue in the thumb hole), or plastic wrap. Again, using a little dollop of lube next to the receiver's skin can improve sensitivity.

5 With latex, don't use mineral oils or any lubricants other than those that are water-based, as they will destroy it. There are alternatives to latex, such as nitrile gloves, and polyurethane condoms.

6 Wash all toys after use, with antiseptic soap and hot water, or follow the instructions that come with the toy.

7 Avoid getting semen, vaginal secretions, blood, or feces on any broken skin: that includes the skin in your mouth. If you're performing oral sex without a barrier, then don't floss or brush your teeth just beforehand. And remember that the herpes sores that appear on lips are directly trans-ferable to genitals. It is best to use a barrier!

8 Always dispose of used barriers safely, and never attempt to reuse them.

9 Eroticize safer sex. It doesn't have to be more difficult or unpleasant than utilizing any other contraceptive methods. Putting on a condom can be fun. Try doing it with your mouth.

An Orgasm Sampler

I feel the sensation of my orgasms up inside me, and all the way out to my outer lips. They're deep, pulsing, throbbing, clenching. They're emotionally overwhelming and all-consuming!

The energy builds in my pelvis, or sometimes throughout my whole body, even my brow furrows. Everything gets pulled in to the point where the energy is pushed outwards, that's the point of orgasm. I most often feel it go out through my feet or straight upwards from my pelvis.

I feel trembly and like I'm headed to a cliff, then I'm lifted up when I come, and float back down when I'm done.

I could be in a life-or-death situation and not stop if I was having an orgasm.

My orgasms are a combination of water waves and electricity. The front of my body feels electrical from my shins up to my face. The rest of my body feels liquid, like waves washing through it. Exquisite is too small a word: I feel like my whole body has been hit with a baseball bat.

I don't have the words for it, except that there is a buildup and then release and that I really enjoy it. Plus there is a lot of variation between orgasms, some even verge on boring but necessary.

Orgasm is like a chord that resonates through my whole being, like total release, total fusion with my partner.

My strongest orgasms feel like I am exploding in a ball of blue light, an intense deep blue. The lesser orgasms are like riding an undulating wave of intensity with blue flashes here and there along the way. The strongest leave me drenched in sweat, heart pounding and exhausted. Even the lesser ones are very exciting.

Orgasms are like rolling waves, sometimes sweet little ones, sometimes crashing thunder. They're about sensitivity, playfulness, love, and open sharing!

There is a feeling of surfacing, emerging (maybe like birth!)

For me, orgasm is a release of tension, especially if I'm masturbating. There are definite muscle contractions, sometimes just a few, sometimes lots and lots that go on for quite a while. A very good orgasm with a partner is just completely overwhelming — I can't even begin to describe it. I can orgasm basically whenever I want to, and sometimes in only a few seconds.

An orgasm feels like being possessed by power, and then being flooded by it or flooding it.

Trying to describe orgasms is really difficult, like trying to describe an acid trip. I usually feel tension building up — a definite tingling or tickling, mainly in the pelvic region, also in my nipples. There's a sense of shortness-of-breath, as though I'm very nervous. At the climax my whole body convulses. It feels like a rush of pleasure and heat starting with my clitoris and rushing quickly through my entire body, something like an electric shock. This happens in several waves with diminishing intensity. The first wave is very intense.

Orgasm is a concentrated buzz that builds to an explosion throughout my body.

Orgasm is an all-encompassing heat that increases in power and depth to an explosive and cleansing release.

Orgasm is electrifying, my body held in position, frozen solid waiting for it to end, pounding, rising, warmth, elation, laughter, wild, crazy, like nothing matters except that one moment, everything else falls away. Swept up and up, a rush to beat all rushes. Trying to hold it, hold on and slowly having it recede to end in calm contentment.

As these lyrical descriptions of orgasm illustrate, women are starting to define their own sexuality and it is wonderful to see us go beyond the limits that have held us in a state of shame. We still have a long way to go to dispel the old damaging ideas about how sex is *meant* to be, but we are finally beginning to celebrate the glory of our bodies' capacities. Put another way, we're having a lot more fun when we're not so desperate to be "normal."

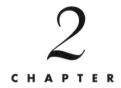

CHAPTER

What Works,
What Doesn't, and Why

The "how" of sex has to do with getting my lover to set the stage, to prepare me emotionally first — to create a sense of safety, slowly, lovingly, attentively, to open me up physically before approaching my genitals.

his chapter is intended to offer pointers on some of the practical aspects of lovemaking, rather than providing a complete guide. There is a great deal to be said that I don't have room to include here. I strongly recommend *The New Good Vibrations Guide to Sex* (Cathy Winks and Anne Semans, Cleis Press) for clear and specific information about the many different ways that we can be sexual.

An Anatomy Review

Sexual responses are as varied as physical appearance, and having an orgasm is by no means all that women need from sex. However, most women want to have an orgasm or two at some point, and many do need specific kinds of stimulation. Some basic information about women's anatomy might help, as well as support my discussions in later chapters.

We are so hung up about and divorced from our bodies in this culture that couples are often too embarrassed to really study one another's bodies, and end up fumbling around in the dark. Unfortunately, the erotic parts of the body don't contain magnets that will automatically draw fingers, tongues, penises, or any other desirable object to them. And fumbling around in the dark doesn't generally lead to a delightfully sensual experience. Given that women's anatomy varies so much, it's a good idea for anyone who is making love to a woman to take the time and trouble to admire what she's got between her legs and familiarize themselves with her physical parts.

Many people assume that female sexual organs consist of the vagina and the clitoris. In fact, the part that is actually visible from the outside is the **vulva**, which is comprised of the **inner** and **outer labia**, the **glans** of the **clitoris**, and the **clitoral hood** (which often obscures the glans until you either pull it back, or become aroused). Even today, girls may grow up in total ignorance of the existence of their clitoris and vagina; in fact, for many girls, it is the use of a tampon that first introduces them to the vagina. But if they ever wash down there then they know what the vulva feels like.

Apart from the fact that knowing what is where greatly facilitates lovemaking, vulvas are beautiful to look at. Sadly, it is not just those who love women who need to learn to love vulvas, it is also the women who own them: many of us are repulsed by our own genitals. How can you experience sex as loving when you feel that way about your sexual parts? There are plenty of ways to go about learning to love yourself. First, familiarize yourself with your own vulva, using a mirror. You can put the mirror on the floor and squat over it, and then pull your lips aside with your fingers to see what's really there. You may also want to check out what you look like when you are aroused because the color and shape can change quite dramatically.

Female genitals vary enormously in size, shape, color, and amount of hair. Familiarizing yourself with other women's genitals will reassure you that yours aren't weird. If you don't want to or aren't able to do this first hand, there are several books with excellent illustrations. The best of these is probably *Femalia* (edited by Joani Blank, published by Down There Press). Others are listed in the Resources.

Knowledge of anatomy also helps to make sense of sexual responses. The clitoris is actually much bigger than the little nub of hard flesh (the glans) that I manipulated to achieve my first orgasm. It consists of hard tissue with legs (or wings, technically referred to as *crura*) that extend into the walls of the vagina, and are surrounded by spongy tissue that swells when a woman is aroused. When the clitoris is erect the glans gets bigger and protrudes from under its hood.

The **perineal sponge** is a pad of spongy erectile tissue that lies between the rectum and the rear wall of the vagina, and the **urethral sponge** is another pad of spongy erectile tissue that lies between the urethral canal (which leads to the bladder) and the front wall of the vagina. They can both be felt through the walls of the vagina and they tend to be the most erotically sensitive parts of it. The part of the urethral sponge that you can feel from inside the vagina is known as the **G spot** or the **G spot prostate**. It is homologous to the male prostate gland and some women find it to be highly sensitive.

The sexual organs are supported by a sling of muscle called the **pubococcygeal**, or **PC, muscle**.

The word clitoris is starting to be used as a catch-all term that refers to all of a woman's sex organs. I think this is a little confusing, but it does help to change the ridiculous perception that female genitalia consist of separate and distinct parts. The whole area is interconnected with an intricate web of muscles, nerves, and blood vessels. When the glans of the clitoris is stimulated, *all* of her erectile tissue, including the urethral sponge and the perineal sponge, will probably swell, and vice versa.

The urethral opening is between the vaginal entrance and the clitoral hood. You can see it if you pull your inner labia apart: it is a small hole, with a slight mound around it. Laura, a nurse, reports that once she had a female patient whose urethral opening was actually inside her vagina and therefore not visible at all. So if your anatomy is different, it doesn't necessarily mean something is wrong.

The urethral opening may be quite sensitive to touch. Many women find it very arousing to be stroked in that area.

The vagina is often thought of as a hole. In fact, the only time it is visible as a hole is when the erectile tissue around the entrance is engorged, which usually happens when a woman is very aroused. At other times the entrance to the vagina may be quite difficult to find. If you're searching in vain for your partner's vagina, it probably means your partner is not yet sufficiently aroused or ready for penetration. Moreover, in its resting state, the vagina is not an empty space. The muscles that form the walls of the vagina lie against each other, so that there is no space between them. As a woman becomes aroused, the muscles contract and pull away from each other, forming a cave.

An Oral Review

Many women find the glans of the clitoris is too sensitive to take any direct touch. You can have plenty of fun stimulating the clitoris in different ways: grasping the shaft between your fingers; stroking the place at the base of the inner lips where the legs of the clitoris lie under the skin; stroking the glans just above or below the hood, or through the labia (which are fairly stretchy). Often there is a very specific spot, usually to one side of the glans, that's more sensitive than any other. Ask!

Using your tongue on any of the same places can be wonderful. Women tend to be paranoid that their lovers don't like going down on them. However, all the men who filled in the men's questionnaire said they did. Here's some responses from a few of them:

It's usually my favorite part of sex.

Oh yes, that's my favorite part, I do that at least 90% of the time.

Very much so, I rarely engage in any sexual activity that doesn't include it.

YES! I do it at least as often as she will let me.

YESSSSSSS!!! I do it as often as I can. God, I do love it.

In spite of these enthusiastic testimonies, many women are not able to enjoy cunnilingus because they are afraid they smell or taste bad. Plenty of unasked-for reassurance from a lover should relieve some of the anxiety. Usually a woman's negative feelings about herself can be traced to having been told that "down there" is "dirty." You can reverse this dreadful piece of conditioning by smelling and tasting yourself after you have had a bath. Slide your finger inside your vagina and then smell and taste your own juices. When you've decided that, after all, it's not so awful, then do the same thing at different times of the day. Try it at different times in your cycle. Women's smells tend to alter throughout the month. Get to know yourself. And remember, even if you decide that you don't particularly like your smell or taste, that doesn't mean your lover will agree with you. Ask.

Every human being has his or her own distinct personal odor, and North Americans tend to have an especially strong paranoia about their body smells. Although we may not be consciously aware of it, personal odor may play an important part in sexual attraction. We all sweat, and we'd be in a sorry state if we didn't, since it is an essential bodily function. You may very well find yourself dripping with sweat during a great sexual encounter. I am certainly not recommending that you abandon good personal hygiene habits, but I am suggesting that if you insist on maintaining ladylike behavior at all times, you may be cheating yourself out of a passionate sexual experience.

Women who have had very negative sexual experiences, whether consciously recalled or not, may always have negative associations with anything that reminds them of sex. The sense of smell is the most primitive of all the senses, which means that it is the one most likely to key into the subconscious, and bring up intense feelings you never knew were there. In other words, if you cannot get over your dislike of the smell of sex, or the smell of your own sexual organs, it may be because the smell triggers some subconscious feelings of abhorrence that are not so much about the smell itself, but about sex. This may be because you've had some very unpleasant experiences around sex or it may be because of the fear and disgust around sex that we inherit from the culture.

The best antidote to that fear and disgust is the experience of enjoyment through sexual stimulation, and well-executed oral stimulation is one of the most reliable ways of experiencing pleasure for most women. But performing oral sex on a woman is not necessarily as easy as you might think. Linda believes that men are misled by pornographic films:

In porn movies they show the actors attacking a woman's vulva, licking just like a cat's tongue in a bowl of milk, I mean that's okay when you are just on the edge of orgasm, but not to start out with!

I asked several women how they would instruct someone to perform oral sex on them. Here are some of their replies:

Play with the tip of my clitoris with the tip of your tongue.

I like oral sex to be fairly gentle; my clitoris is really sensitive. I want to feel that slickness.

I can only come with oral stimulation. I want him to suck and bite my clit a lot.

I like my clitoris to be licked, usually gently at first, but then with varying degrees of pressure and speed. I prefer one or two fingers inside me later on in the process. I don't really like having the rest of my vulva licked, or a tongue inside my vagina, or my clitoris being sucked. (And definitely no teeth!)

I guess I would tell her to give me a long, slow, gentle kiss, pretending my clit was her tongue. Then when I'm about to come, I like to be slowly entered with a finger or two.

Use the tip of your tongue really lightly and slowly around and on my clit. I always want it done rhythmically; find one rhythm and don't change it.

I want my partner to start by kissing my belly, working down to my pussy. Then s/he should lightly run the tip of his/her tongue from my anus to the top of my clit, teasing me. Then s/he should stick his/her tongue in my vagina deep and hard, before moving up to my clit. I like having my clit licked, kissed, bitten gently, and manually stroked while fingers explore my G spot and my anus. I also like to know that my partner enjoys what s/he is doing; verbal acknowledgement is great and turns me on even more.

Some women stress the importance of rhythm and speed.

I want my clitoris stimulated gently and rhythmically while she's talking dirty to me and penetrating my vagina deeply and slowly and rhythmically.

I need a gradual rhythmic increase in speed and pressure on my clit.

Sometimes it takes perseverance.

I only have clitoral orgasms from using my own hand or from someone going down on me. Some of my lovers haven't been willing to stay down long enough — it usually takes fifteen or twenty minutes. Not everyone does it right, and I'm shy about asking for what I want.

There is a small percentage of women who aren't turned on by oral sex, so be sure to ask first.

Clitoral stimulation by another person just doesn't seem to work all that well. I find receiving oral sex to be frustrating and somewhat boring, because no matter how intense it is, I never really come from it. Manual stimulation of my clit is actually an impediment to orgasm, strangely enough.

I need my clitoris to be stimulated by hand; oral stimulation mostly doesn't work for me. It has to be very direct and at first fairly hard stimulation, lighter as I get closer to orgasm. I orgasm more easily if my nipples are being stimulated at the same time as my clitoris.

Penetration

You may very well find that those who don't like oral sex really enjoy penetration. Chapter Eleven is all about penetration, but here are a few pointers. It is common to want slow penetration combined with clitoral stimulation.

I find that I must have my clitoris stimulated in order to reach orgasm, but the orgasms are deeper if I am also penetrated vaginally.

I need penetration and clitoral stimulation.

I orgasm most often when my clit is being stimulated orally and when I'm being penetrated anally. I orgasm best when I am slowly worked towards a climax.

The sensations of penetration vary greatly, depending on how excited the woman is; what she is being penetrated with; whether it is being held still or moved around; whether it's curved or straight; how it's being moved (in and out, round and round, slow or fast, long deep strokes or short ones, all the way out or not quite); and at what angle it is being held. It can be very exciting to be penetrated with something as small as a finger if the finger is doing the right thing, which, again, varies from woman to woman. A few women might always want to be filled up with something large. The shape of the object makes a big difference too. If it gets bigger towards the base it may be more uncomfortable. But some women like a bigger base.

A Different Kind of Blow Job

Another technique that works for some women is blowing on the genital area. This provides a pleasant tickling effect. Try putting your lips around the clitoris or the labia and "buzzing" with them. Also try having a hot cup of tea or some other liquid nearby; take a mouthful, hold it, and then dribble it slowly over her clitoral area or squirt it into her vagina. (Yes, it'll make the bed wet, so what?) You can try the same thing with cold water or chunks of ice, but be careful — I have found that ice on my genital area is painful and makes me tighten up, whereas heat feels glorious and makes me relax.

How to Ask

The personal accounts that appear throughout the book paint a very varied picture of what women like. So don't use the same formula on everyone. Each partner is an individual. Ask her what she wants. Of course, this isn't always as easy as it seems. A number of men pointed out in their questionnaires that it sometimes feels tacky to ask, "Did you come?" But there are plenty of other ways to find out if your partner had a good time. Try, "Would you have preferred to stop sooner than we did?" Or, "Would you like to have gone on longer?" What follows is a list of questions for partners to ask after a lovemaking session, that most women find relatively easy to respond to:

- Was my rhythm too fast/slow/irregular?
- Would you have liked me to stay longer on your clitoris?
- Was I in the right spot?
- Would you have liked more general or more specific stimulation?
- Did I use enough lube?
- Did I enter you too soon or would you have liked me inside you earlier?
- Do you like trying different positions, and if so, which?
- Would you have liked me to use something else inside you?
- What other ways would you like me to touch you another time, that I didn't this time?
- Were there ways you would have liked to touch me?

If you are a woman who wants to ask for these things, you can turn them around and say:

- I tend to have even stronger orgasms when . . .
- You can make me come very quickly if you . . .
- I loved it when you . . . , and you could have done that for longer.
- Would it have been okay with you if I had put my hand on my clit/used a vibrator/asked you to go down on me/slowed you down/ asked you to stop?
- Do you like to use your fingers inside a woman? Let me show you the most sensitive part of my vagina.

Or any other tactful way of suggesting that you could have even more fun next time. In my opinion it is always best to get suggestive from the beginning of the relationship; otherwise you could get stuck in a monotonous routine, and it becomes a very big deal to change.

One creative way to get a clear picture of what excites your partner is to have her or him literally draw a diagram of their arousal. The two drawings on the next page are by Jesse and myself. Mine represents a masturbation session; in hers, I am the doer and she is the receiver. Fifteen minutes into it I answered the telephone and had a ten-minute conversation about gardening. As you can see, this interruption did not curtail Jesse's arousal, even though I paid her little attention while I was on the phone.

Masturbation

The vast majority of women and men have their first orgasms through masturbating, and some women only come through

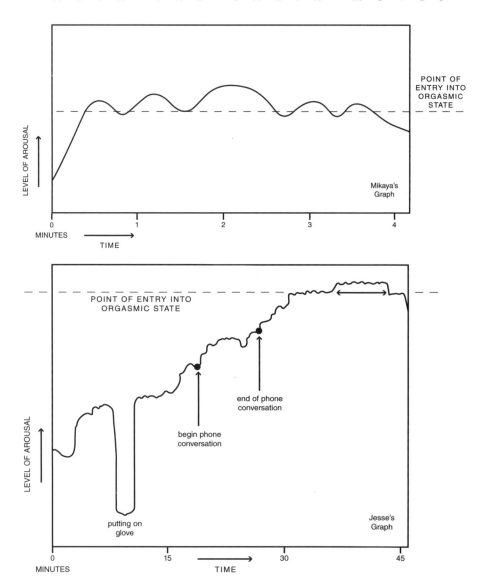

POINT OF
ENTRY INTO
ORGASMIC
STATE

LEVEL OF AROUSAL

Mikaya's
Graph

0   1   2   3   4

MINUTES

TIME

POINT OF ENTRY INTO
ORGASMIC STATE

end of phone
conversation

begin phone
conversation

LEVEL OF AROUSAL

putting on
glove

Jesse's
Graph

0   15   30   45

MINUTES

TIME

masturbation. I strongly recommend that all women learn about pleasuring themselves. There are lots of good reasons for masturbating. It can be a great way to reverse any negative messages we may have about sex, and about our bodies.

It is also wonderful to find out how much pleasure you can experience without being dependent on someone else. Getting to know your own body is liberating and empowering, and can be a great help in achieving sexual pleasure with a partner. Not only is it a source of enjoyment, it can increase your self-confidence, and it costs nothing. It can also be a straightforward and effective way to release tension.

Alas, we live in a society that is loaded with taboos about masturbation. Earlier this century, it was still thought to be responsible for making women hysterical, and surgical removal of the clitoris and the outer lips was sometimes undertaken to remedy the "problem." Women occasionally think that their labia look strange or abnormal, and imagine this to be the result of masturbation. In fact, some women simply happen to have labia that are long or uneven. You are not going to physically alter anything down there by masturbating. Nor will you grow hair on your palms, nor will you go blind, nor will you get addicted. Self-pleasuring is a perfectly natural pastime. Young babies have been observed rocking themselves to orgasm. All of us would probably indulge in it if we weren't trained not to. **There is absolutely no known harm that can come to you through masturbation**, except for the damage that is inflicted on our psyches by an uptight society.

Having said all that, it's still true that many women just can't bring themselves to relax into the joy of self-stimulation.

I do try to masturbate from time to time, especially in the bath. It seems hard to get any satisfaction; I can feel myself coming and enjoy it but I can end up feeling frustrated.

49

Touching myself just didn't feel good to me.

Sometimes it's a very poor second to having a partner, and may even make us more aware that we are alone.

Sometimes masturbating makes me cry and feel exceedingly lonely!

Some women masturbate every day or more, others only masturbate once or twice a month. How much a woman masturbates will probably vary throughout her life, depending on whether she's with a partner, what her general health is like, what else is going on in her life, what her hormones are doing. Most people masturbate because they want an orgasm, but that's not always the case. Since Rita doesn't orgasm, I asked her what she gets out of masturbating:

I like the sensations. I find it cool that my body can do that, can get aroused and feel things.

Clara, who had her first orgasm when she was forty-one, says she used to masturbate in phases as a teenager, usually in the bathroom, since her sexual desire was often connected with the sensation of peeing.

I'd get this intense, acute feeling in my clitoris, and I'd masturbate to relieve it. Sometimes it got rid of the feeling and sometimes it didn't.

The kinds of orgasm a woman experiences through masturbation may be quite different from the kind she has with a partner.

When I'm masturbating I have intense but more localized and shorter orgasms.

There are many different ways to masturbate and many different things to masturbate with. You don't have to be on your own to masturbate: it can be exciting and very satisfying with a partner.

I am in an eight-year monogamous relationship with a woman. After an exchange of "foreplay," stroking and whatever, we masturbate to orgasm at the same time, together. We find this very satisfying. Our relationship is based on mutual interests, sharing, and support, rather than on sex. It wasn't until we were in our forties that we had the emotional maturity to consider sex in other than conventional ways.

I've used my hand, a vibrator, and water pressure to masturbate with. When I'm masturbating, I need to fantasize to come unless my partner is stimulating me by touching my breasts.

Vibrators

Vibrators can be a quick and easy way to give yourself or someone else an orgasm. Even if you come reliably other ways, you may find yourself having a new and different kind of orgasm with a vibrator.

Using a vibrator makes an orgasm inescapable, which is the greatest. I love to feel like an orgasm is coming to get me — no pun intended.

I rarely achieve an orgasm without using my vibrator.

When I masturbate, the direct route is a good quality AC-powered vibrator applied directly to my clit with a great deal of stimulation. There's no subtlety here at all, just sheer intensity.

I had my first orgasm when I was eighteen and I'd just bought a vibrator, one of those cheesy battery-powered ones. It took me maybe two minutes to have my very first orgasm and I was thrilled. I went through several sets of batteries and two vibrators in the next few weeks.

It is very important to realize that different kinds of vibrators, even if they seem to have similar kinds of vibration, can have very different effects. Some just make me numb, so that I can't come from any kind of stimulation after a few minutes of use. It's frustrating and not particularly pleasant. Be prepared to try more than one brand. The smaller, cheaper, battery-powered models may never bring on an orgasm by themselves, but they can be great as an addition to other kinds of stimulation. Various attachments are available to put on the end of a vibrator for anal or vaginal penetration.

But plenty of people don't like them:

Vibrators are too intense, too noisy, and physically irritating.

I tried a vibrator once and found it completely uninteresting.

Many women find their bodies are a lot readier for orgasm when they haven't had one in a while.

It helps if I haven't had sex for a month or so.

But most women report that the more accustomed they are to having orgasms, the more easily they have them.

Sex is like chocolate — the more you have, the more you want.

Emotional Erogenous Zones

Being in love and feeling attracted to our partners are considered important elements of orgasm. And sometimes our feelings for a partner can preclude the need to come.

I usually expect to experience orgasm when I'm with someone, but I'm not attached because I can bring myself to orgasm later if needed. It's the connection that's more important.

Lots of things bring me to orgasm, but my most pleasurable and intense orgasmic experiences happen when I feel emotionally close and connected with my lover: when everything is flowing harmoniously between us, allowing us to open up to deeper and more sensual physical pleasure, including orgasm.

If I'm feeling good and am very attracted to my partner, then I have intense multiple orgasms.

It helps if I trust my partner and am not withholding emotions like anger.

I come most easily when I'm in love.

Some women made it clear that they don't have to know their partners well, or that sex is even hotter when the partner is new.

The sex is usually better if I'm in love and lust with the woman, but I have had big orgasms with women in the past who I didn't fancy but who really touched the right points in me.

Deep love and trust mean I'm more likely to experience intense orgasms, as does that kind of wild sexual chemistry I experience with some women, whether I've just met them or known them a long time.

Several women said that the experience of the lover, and his or her ability to communicate, counts for a lot.

I am most likely to orgasm when my partner is an experienced lovemaker who knows a woman's body and listens to what I tell him, not someone who simply assumes that he knows what will please me because it is what pleased other women.

I like to be teased.

Words help too, to be told I'm gorgeous, that various parts of me are beautiful.

I orgasm when I surrender to the experience.

A number of women stressed the importance of being relaxed and comfortable.

When I'm relaxed and don't have a lot on my mind, I can definitely come more easily.

Some women need complete privacy and assurance that they won't be disturbed.

I need to be assured that no one besides my partner can hear me or know I'm being sexual.

Many women have told me that what never fails to excite them is feeling and seeing their partner's excitement.

In order for me to orgasm, I need to know my partner is excited.

Laughter is an ingredient that makes everything taste better.

I find humor to be a part of the turn-on. Much more memorable and erotic than just good technique.

Some women need to be allowed or need to allow themselves to fantasize.

I need some level of power play between my partner and myself.

I orgasm most easily if I allow myself to fantasize about being "overtaken" by animals.

Physics

Almost any part of the body can be erotically sensitive if it is given attention. Sensuality is an aspect of sexuality, and any sexual encounter can be enhanced by keying into sensual desire. In particular, many women have extremely sensitive nipples.

I can orgasm just from having my nipples touched and stroked, then sucked intensely.

I had a very intense orgasm once when my clitoris, my vagina, and my toes were all being stimulated simultaneously.

Some women need to have their bodies in particular positions.

I come with my legs open, having my clitoris touched. I must be relaxed and free of stress.

I like to be on my knees or to have my legs bent and my body at ninety degrees to my legs.

I can orgasm standing, sitting, lying on my side, or on my back or my front, but I nearly always want my legs closed together.

I must have my legs stretched out to come.

My orgasms are intensified when I am physically restrained or imagining that I am.

Although many women said that they need a slow and powerful lead-in to a climax, good orgasms don't necessarily arise from a stunning buildup.

My partner and I generally have very good orgasms but pretty pedestrian sex. We do the same things most of the time — cud-

dling, kissing, and playing first, followed by penetration with him on top, then turning on our sides with him rubbing his penis against my clitoris until I reach climax. Then we move back to the man-on-top position that he likes best until he reaches climax. I sometimes have a second orgasm then. We don't vary this routine too much because it works well. Whenever we try a different technique it usually turns out to be less satisfactory.

Many women report that they cannot come without using either their own hand or a vibrator, and this often causes them angst when they are with a lover, even though it's not at all unusual.

I need clitoral stimulation from my fingers and/or a vibrator "driven" by me, plus vaginal intercourse.

Thanks to the variations in female anatomy, there are some women who get as much stimulation as they want from their lover's body rubbing on the clitoris while his penis is inside her.

I am most likely to come from intercourse with a man; clitoral stimulation is pretty dicey and usually not that much fun for me when someone else is doing it.

But, in general, the best position for a woman during intercourse is when she is on top, allowing her to situate herself so that she gets exactly the right amount of pressure on her clitoris, and giving her control of the angle and speed of stimulation.

I found that the only way I've ever orgasmed is if I'm on top of my partner with him penetrating my vagina.

I'm more likely to come during intercourse if I'm on top, as if that position is physiologically more conducive to orgasms.

When a woman is on top she may also touch her own clitoris quite easily. And the same goes for lying side-by-side.

Lots and lots of women do not come from vaginal stimulation alone. Clitoral stimulation certainly sweeps the board as the primary method of coming, whether it's done by the woman herself or by her lover, whether it's before, during, or after penetration.

I have clitoral orgasms from consistent stimulation, oral or manual, to the area around the clitoris. It must be lubricated, and preferably some variation in pace and type of stimulation with more rapid stimulation as orgasm becomes imminent.

I want a rapid back-and-forth stimulation (manual or oral) of my clitoris, starting slowly, with increasing speed and pressure. Actually, as I consider it, not so directly on the clitoris but sort of at the top of the clitoral shaft.

I like my clitoris stroked gently when I am well on my way to orgasm.

I have big orgasms, usually from oral sex, that are very intense, last longer, and involve a full body shudder.

I usually come from receiving oral sex, combined with anal or vaginal stimulation.

One Is Not Always Enough

You might take note that just because a woman orgasms once doesn't necessarily mean she is done.

I like penetration for a good long time if I'm in the mood, but my lover tends to want to join in with her orgasm after a while, so even though I experience orgasm I often feel it could be taken a lot further.

Clitoral stimulation can lead to orgasm without ejaculation. Then sometimes further stimulation leads to ejaculation and total release.

I do relish the caring and persistent and clever lover whose activities produce successive orgasmic waves.

Tuning In and Turning On

For many of us, what's happening on a psychic and emotional level is very important. This is really what foreplay means to women: taking the time to experience and build the energy on all levels, not just the physical.

It may be that sex is not so much a body thing for me, so what someone does to me is not necessarily very important as long as their intentions are good.

Sex for me is about union and connection and power exchange.

Sex is not merely genital, but energetic: the whole person is involved, not just a bundle of nerve endings.

I find the pacing, the arousal in tandem with my lover, the gestures and courtship (from romantic to dirty) to be essential. Lots and lots and lots of foreplay, all day, all week, words, gestures, one finger touching one place.

Being tuned in to your lover is vital. I have only had one lover who could reliably make me come with her hand. When I asked her what her secret was, she said: "Somehow

I plug into your experience so that I experience what I am doing to you as though I were you."

And being tuned in to your own body is just as important. Anna Marti says:

For me the challenge is to daily inhabit my body in ways that I become totally engaged, whether working, eating, loving, or playing, because the erotic experience truly is about every cell in my body becoming involved, directing my mind and my heart so that my body may become involved; the sexual, creative, ecstatic cells are not solely located in the genitals.

If you manage all this, maybe you will have orgasms like these:

Quite often during clitoral stimulation it will feel as if my partner has just found a particular spot that pierces up through me, which then sets off waves rolling down on me (I don't know what the waves are — sort of like warm internal strokes). An intense orgasm will combine these physical waves with waves of emotion, and very occasionally these will be strong enough to make me cry. When the clitoral situation is combined with penetration, the orgasm is more about a sense of completion and wholeness.

I can lose myself completely in a powerful orgasm. It's like being ripped out from inside. It's like planets colliding. Yes, the earth moves, but not before the Milky Way dissolves.

3

CHAPTER

The Physical Experience of Orgasm

I think the main difference in the types of orgasm I have has to do with how involved I feel. I can have orgasms from clitoral stimulation which just feel like physical buildup and release (also true of masturbation even when it involves penetration). These orgasms generally feel confined to my genital area. Orgasms induced by my partner licking, stroking, and penetrating me, I feel through my whole body, and they are likely to have a stronger emotional component. They are the sort that leave me feeling more cleansed and released. Sometimes I'll have an orgasm while making love to someone else from rubbing against them or hearing them. They usually feel like a sort of fizz up through my body and they're physical rather than emotional (although, of course, they have power/excitement connotations).

When I have multiple orgasms they are a mixture of types, for instance, a couple of little ones followed by a big "emotional" one or vice versa.

I have unlimited types of orgasm: sometimes they involve the whole of me, sometimes just specific parts. The most wonderful ones are when each one of my muscles tightens and then releases.

60

Each orgasm is different — some give merely physical release; some are spiritual ecstasy. At its best, there is a slow exquisite buildup that feels increasingly electrical, where gradually more and more parts of my body get "involved" in the buildup, where I begin to feel down to the cells of my body, and up to the spirit of my heart, like a whirlpool that spins wider and deeper.

When I first began asking women to explain what exactly went on for them when they were being sexual, many had very little to say. They didn't have the language to describe their feelings and sensations. But as the interviews progressed, their words started to flow. In the end, everyone said they found it fascinating to think and talk about in depth, especially when they had the opportunity to listen to other women.

It's not surprising that finding the words to describe an orgasm is initially difficult, because we have been trained to avoid thinking about our bodies and our feelings. In fact we are trained *not* to verbalize our sexual experiences at all. Thus it is initially uncomfortable to try to bring our sexual feelings into the mental realm: we would often prefer to keep them unfocused, blurry. A great deal of the feedback I got from the questionnaire was embarrassment. Some women dismissed it, saying, "Oh, there's already been so much written about sex." Others openly acknowledged that they didn't even want to read through the questionnaire because it made them think about sex more than they liked to. In many cases it was clear that the discomfort went as far as real shame. Apparently the sex-negative attitudes of our society extend even to *thinking* about sex.

The Myth of the Definitive Orgasm

Freud defined two types of female orgasm: vaginal and clitoral. He claimed that as a woman matured, she would — or *should* — transfer the site of her orgasm to the vagina. In other words, she should experience orgasm as a result of intercourse, and not as a result of clitoral stimulation. What we must remember is that Freud was only relaying what the men of his time wanted to believe. They didn't want to hear that intercourse is only one form of sexual play and that most women prefer a variety. They didn't want to be responsible for their partner's pleasure. They just wanted to hear that it was their job to get on top and pump away until they themselves came, and if the woman didn't come in that time, she was inadequate, and it certainly wasn't a male's responsibility to do anything differently.

Although many of the women I spoke with certainly experience intense pleasure from vaginal penetration, relatively few come without clitoral stimulation. They say either that they have lots of different kinds of orgasm, or only one kind; or that the difference is not in where the orgasm originates, but in its intensity; or that they like to have vaginal stimulation when they are having a "clitoral" orgasm; or that they need to have clitoral stimulation in order to have a "vaginal" orgasm. Many said they could not equate their experience of orgasm with what was being done to them, because there were far too many other factors involved. Some had their own classifications that had nothing to do with clitoral or vaginal categories.

I have two different kinds of orgasm. One is created by tension and the other is more relaxed. The tension type are more electrical; the relaxed ones are like riding a wave.

Mine vary. Some are quiet as a sigh. Some are tumultuous — a tension building, pure delight, anticipation, everything concentrated upon sensation, and then waves of release, pleasure, joy — and then, a new tension, a new peak, total incandescent energy.

In other words, a strict separation into vaginal and clitoral is an artificial and very misleading division, imposed from a male perspective. However, it is a classification that has been widely used, and the clitoris and the vagina are *the* two areas of female anatomy that have been identified as the centers of erotic sensation. I believe it is a mistake to think of the vagina as one organ and the clitoris as another separate organ. They are parts of the same structure.

Most women I interviewed were rather vague when I asked if they had separate vaginal and clitoral orgasms, and I had to ask several times; even then the clearest distinction I got was usually very qualified. Women on the verge of orgasm are often experiencing diffuse sensations that permeate their whole genital area and sometimes their whole body. And they may react quite differently to the same stimuli from one day to the next, depending on many variables, such as who is touching them and what with, or the time of the month, or how relaxed they were prior to being sexual.

I don't have one sensation of orgasm but many, depending on many things: whether it's the first or the twenty-fifth, whether I relax and let the sensations just roll over me, what kind of lead-in there is, if it's just purely a physical response, and so on.

Different things cause different orgasms — an intense vibrator can cause an explosive one whereas a timid, battery-operated vibrator will make an irritatingly fluttery and less-than-complete feeling.

The most common kind of orgasms I have are several little clitoral/vaginal pulsating ones in a row. With penetration I have a deep orgasm that involves uterine contractions. Multiple orgasms are like little shuddering quakes.

I like to have fast, hard orgasms during my period to relieve my cramps. If I'm masturbating (which I do most every day) and I'm tired then it usually takes a lot of buildup and I have one or two big spasms. I have long orgasms with my partner — they feel deep (even without penetration), they last a long time, and they make me shiver for several minutes afterwards.

Women who do not come easily are much more likely to be able to be specific about what they need, but they're also unlikely to identify with the separation between clitoral and vaginal orgasms.

Of the women I have personally been sexual with, there is one woman who came close to fitting the pattern of having truly distinct vaginal and clitoral orgasms. (*None* of the women I spoke with related to the value judgement that women should cease to have clitoral orgasms as they matured.) Judy's orgasms are clearly defined: one comes from clitoral stimulation only, and the other comes from vaginal stimulation only, and the sensations associated with each one are quite distinct. What is interesting about her sexual responses is that, because she has such distinct vaginal and clitoral orgasms, and never mixes the two kinds of stimulation, her descriptions of them are very articulate, whereas none of the other women I spoke to could separate them with such precision. Even women who did define separate kinds of orgasm were rarely able to say categorically what kind of stimulation would lead to which kind of orgasm. Judy's unswerving clarity about this was unique among the women I interviewed.

I have a clitoral orgasm either from having oral sex performed on me, or from using my hand on my clitoris. I don't want penetration when I'm having my clitoris stimulated: I find it distracting and not particularly pleasant. This kind of orgasm racks my body, it pulls me forward, and keeps coming in a series of waves. My abdominal muscles spasm, curling me up, pulling me in. I feel lines of electricity running down my legs, and into my abdomen and chest. The energy feels very central, like a core inside me, and from there it spreads to different parts of my body. After one clitoral orgasm my clit is way too sensitive to be touched any more, so I have one big one, and that's it.

Vaginal orgasms are a going-out energy; they feel like an expulsive thing. I'm so into the sensation of penetration that I want my lover to concentrate all her energy on that, and I don't really want her to touch my clitoris. My vaginal orgasms are multiple, and each succeeding one gets more intense as I have them, until my whole body shudders and vibrates, from my head down to my feet or my feet up to my head. How many I have depends on my lover's stamina. I'm not sure how many I can have, maybe up to ten.

A clitoral orgasm has a mental connection. I have to feel an element of safety and vulnerability. I can't let my body go in the same way, like I can with a vaginal orgasm. I can't be disconnected. I need my head and my heart involved. With vaginal orgasms, sometimes just my body is involved, my entire body, outside as well as inside. They are coarser, more external, more flesh and blood, more body, less energetic.

Carol is fairly typical of many women: although she enjoys both kinds of stimulation, she's not able to be specific about what would make one or the other kind of orgasm occur:

I definitely have different kinds, and I guess I'd divide them into vaginal and clitoral. But I always have to have some kind of clitoral stimulation, even for a vaginal orgasm. These are more emotional and intense, they are deep, constricting, pounding. I feel the contractions far inside. The waves from one orgasm can go on for more than a minute sometimes, and then I can have another one, often five or six. The second one is always stronger than the first. I can sometimes have these without penetration, just from long, hard clitoral stimulation. But if I'm being penetrated, I'm sure to have a vaginal orgasm. The clitoral orgasms are sort of an electrical jolt, and sometimes they're just like a blip. They're more a surface experience.

Victoria craves deep penetration and she corroborates Carol's experience of "blips," although she has a different name for them:

I've tried to like vibrators, but I just don't. My orgasms are not nearly as powerful with them, just this quick "veeet!"

Donna, like Carol, differentiates between clitoral and vaginal orgasms, and her vaginal orgasms are multiple, but otherwise her description of what she experiences is quite different; her clitoral orgasms are more physical and much shorter:

I have very different kinds of orgasms: I guess you could call them clitoral and vaginal. Clitoral orgasms are fast and hard, intense and short, more physical. I tend to hold my breath with them. Vaginal orgasms have more of a buildup and there's a sense of pulsing, which I think is a uterine contraction, although sometimes it's a whole-body contraction if the orgasm is more extended. I get aftershocks as well. Over several hours, they may vary a great deal. They may occur in different parts of my body, depending on what's being stimulated. All the parts of my body are sensual. I can feel orgasms from the back of my throat all the way down to my vagina, and in my legs.

Andrea is typical of the many women who aren't able to make specific distinctions all the time, but she talks of clitoral orgasms as being more final:

Although my vaginal and clitoral orgasms are not always distinctly separate, sometimes I have a vaginal orgasm when my clitoris is not even awake. My clitoral orgasms are not generally multiple, but my vaginal orgasms are countless. I just fly for hours sometimes, coming over and over and over. I like to make love till I'm exhausted, and then have one big clitoral orgasm and stop. Otherwise I wouldn't know when to stop. With a clitoral one, I hold my breath tightly, and then I scream. With vaginal ones I pant a lot and breathe very deeply.

Other women agree that a clitoral orgasm is more fulfilling. But Linci relates that the orgasms she has that involve penetration are often more powerful:

My clitoral orgasms are quick: they take the edge off, they're easy physical manipulation. Throbbing orgasms are the deepest and most intense; they're shocking. I can feel my lips ringing with the throbbing. I feel like I'm totally tripping, and I have these circulatory pulsations that go on for two or three minutes. These orgasms go on so long, they're almost continuous, I'm so totally in it. I have to have penetration in order to experience a throbber, but it doesn't have to be deep penetration.

Beyond Vaginal and Clitoral

Dee has classified her orgasms according to her very own system, which has nothing to do with whether they are clitoral or vaginal. This was her very prompt response when I asked her if she had separate kinds of orgasms:

I have three kinds of orgasm. One I call the waterfall*: it's like a whooshing out and down; the sensation goes up to my waist and then shoots downwards out of my toes. Then there's the* sparkler*: that's like a sparkler, you know, fireworks. It emanates from my lower belly and sends sprinklies out every-where, sideways as well as up and down. It's very white. Then there's one I call* Saturn*, because I feel like that's where I go. I don't have them so often, but when I do they are really exquis-ite. I feel them in my whole body from my head to my toes.*

I nearly always have at least four orgasms at one time, and the fourth is always the best. When I have a Saturn, it's always the fourth.

Dee loves penetration, but does not generally come with-out some kind of clitoral stimulation, even if it's fairly indirect. She didn't relate her different kinds of orgasm to what was being done to her so much as to her emotional state, and she said she rarely or never could project in advance which kind she was likely to have.

Dee's desire to have direct stimulation on her clitoris, at the same time as vaginal penetration, is very common. Not many women say they are able to come from vaginal pene-tration alone. What makes one woman able to do this when others can't? It might be simply physical. In 1958, Dr. Kermit Krantz performed several autopsies on women and went to the trouble of counting the nerve endings in the pelvic area. He discovered quite enough variation in the distribution of the nerves to account for differing sexual responses. (*The Classic Clitoris: Historic Contributions to Scientific Sexuality*, Thomas Power Lowry, editor, Nelson-Hall, Chicago, copyright 1978. K. E. Krantz, Innervation of the human vulva and vagina, *Obstetrics and Gynecology*, 12: 382-396).

But, most likely, it is a combination of physical factors and cultural conditioning from a society that has trained women to rein in their passion. I have attempted to address some of these issues in later chapters.

Following my initial series of interviews, I identified several categories of orgasms, and I fed these categories back to the women I was interviewing. Here are some of the labels I assigned:

- flying orgasms
- wave orgasms
- falling orgasms
- pounding orgasms
- surface orgasms
- deep orgasms
- disappearing orgasms
- crying orgasms
- throbbers
- veets
- blips

These labels were the ones that generally received the most positive response from women (such as, "Yes, I think that describes what I experience.") However, they are quite arbitrary, because I invented them only as a way of encouraging women to form words to describe their orgasms. And for every woman who told me that one or more of those particular words did describe her experience, there were other women who said, "No, I wouldn't use that word." You may recognize some of these categories in the following descriptions.

I wondered if women like Dee, who define their orgasms very clearly, do so because they have been mostly with one lover, and therefore tend to stick to one particular kind of lovemaking. Dee has been monogamous for twenty years. Perhaps women who have had more lovers are more likely to have different kinds of orgasm, and have a harder time defining them. But every time I form a theory about women and their orgasms, someone pops up to disprove it. Jan has had many lovers, but only has one type of orgasm.

I always assumed my orgasms were clitoral, because I have to have my clitoris stimulated to come. Then I heard people talking about a whole-body orgasm and I realized that that is what I have: my whole body is completely involved in coming. Every muscle in my body takes part in the buildup; it's like the energy has to align itself in my limbs and in my head and neck; I have to stretch out my toes, and clench my fists, and straighten my arms and legs. And when I do all that, when I have made my body into the right kind of container, then the movement of whatever it is on my clitoris takes wing and I fly like an arrow, I shoot outwards, and the energy surges outwards in a huge wave of light, and I'm carried on that crest of energy until I fly down the other side and there I am, all vibrating and renewed, washed clean by the energy that carried me. And then it picks me up again, and off we go, three, four, five, six or more times. The first time is often an effort — I have to really work at getting my body into alignment, at opening up the channels the energy flows through, but then the second time all the doors are already open and I just fly with it. I just soar up and over. It's delightful. My whole body glows, like a light bulb. My clitoris is the filament, but light comes from the whole bulb, which is my whole body.

Jan says she has to have firm and regular stimulation on her clitoris in order to come, and although she doesn't *have* to have penetration, it really helps her to have a powerful orgasm. Clara is similar to Jan: she doesn't relate to having more than one kind, and she has to have her clitoris stimulated very exactly with a vibrator. Unlike Jan, she's not interested in being penetrated when she comes:

The best orgasms start very much around my clitoris. The buildup is exquisite, and it's part of the orgasm. The anticipatory tension is all consuming, as my whole being is focused on that one goal. I feel this huge tension in my thighs. Then the tension peaks and I'm riding the wave. I feel the energy deep in my womb, then it floods down my legs and up into my belly.

Like Dee, Jesse cannot tell what sparks off a particular kind. She has a number of different orgasms and I refer to some of them in other parts of the book. Here's how she defines a couple of the more unusual (and difficult) kinds:

I occasionally have disappearing orgasms: the whole buildup feels like it'll be a normal orgasm and then it's over without any release, no fireworks at the top. It may be that those are one-contraction orgasms versus what normally might be dozens, though I don't think I'm aware of the contractions as discrete events until the main part's over, and I'm having aftershocks. Maybe it's just that my body is not able to maintain and accumulate enough charge at those times and that's why they disappear.

Sometimes I have crying orgasms, like the sweetest liquid emotional pain wells up to my chest and throat, and crying and coming are the same thing — they're indistinguishable.

Jean rarely comes without using a vibrator on her clitoris, but she relates that she has three distinct kinds of orgasm (although she also said she wasn't sure that they all qualified as such):

One is from using my vibrator directly on my clitoris, although I may often have something inside me as well. These are like going over a mountain, or riding a wave. Then there are ones that I have when someone is sucking on some part of me, such as my fingers, or my toes maybe, or my dildo if I'm wearing one, and there is some clitoral stimulation as well. Those feel like a shooting outward. I get this rushing feeling in my body. The end of the orgasm isn't the same as the first one I described. It's more like a dissipation than a complete release, leaving some tension behind. The third kind usually happens if I've been doing a lot of foreplay, and I have a strong emotional bond with my lover. These are electrical and they go through my head, taking my head off.

Maluma only relates to one kind of orgasm, although she can have it from penetration alone, or from clitoral stimulation, or from making love to someone else.

There's a building up and a letting go at the same time, right around my clitoris. It builds and builds, and then I get the "it's gonna happen" feeling. I get tingleys in my clitoris, and then bigger feelings that go into my belly, and then those feelings rise up and go downwards at the same time. The really good orgasms go up through my heart and out of the top of my head. It's like I am the wave, not someone riding it. I used to only have two or three at a time, but now I have five or six.

Betty also has only one kind of orgasm. She needs clitoral stimulation to come, although she also enjoys penetration, separately or simultaneously. She has one big one and that's it — she doesn't want to be touched any more.

My orgasms are like an earthquake or an explosion; they explode out of me. They are a deep, pounding, clenching petit mort that radiates from my entire pelvis up and down my body in shock waves. They're like a seizure; they pick me up and throw me around. I can't imagine having more than one.

Laura doesn't particularly enjoy clitoral stimulation, and would never seek it out. But she loves penetration and comes copiously.

I wouldn't use the words exquisite or clenching or pounding or electrical. Maybe riding a wave. I feel it all over my body, especially in my lower belly. I get goosebumps on my head and neck. I ejaculate a lot, which embarrasses me. I normally have probably five to seven, and the third and fourth are the strongest.

By all accounts only one factor seems to be consistent: women who relate to the distinction between vaginal and clitoral say that they tend to hold their breath when they are working up to a clitoral orgasm.

Combination Orgasms

An orgasm that occurs as a result of simultaneous vaginal and clitoral stimulation might be considered a combination orgasm. Wouldn't it seem logical that this would be best of all? Surprisingly enough, not many women related to combinations, and those who did presented conflicting views about them.

I have two kinds: the clitoral ones feel like the epicenter is my clitoris, whereas the focus of an orgasm when I'm being penetrated is all inside, quite different from a clitoral orgasm. When I'm being penetrated there is a big buildup and then a release. Everything stops at the peak. I don't like to mix the two too much. One is always more dominant.

For a clitoral orgasm, I absolutely need direct clitoral stimulation. A clitoral orgasm has a slower buildup. I get more tense leading up to clitoral orgasms. I hold my breath, and it's a very long come, but not multiple. It can last half an hour or so. It's a bit like flying, and it's very much a wave.

I have vaginal orgasms without any clitoral stimulation. They're localized and I'm more likely to have them when I'm feeling relaxed. They're in my first and second chakra, and they're multiple. Combination orgasms are not multiple — they are like one big clitoral orgasm with a vaginal orgasm at the same time.

A combination orgasm is an all-encompassing experience. It builds, then goes down, then up. It doesn't go out my feet. In fact, it doesn't go anywhere, it comes! I don't really want to call it energy — it's more like power, and it feels very active, the way it surges down my legs.

Surface versus Depth

For most women, it seems that the primary variation in orgasms is in their intensity, and how much the orgasm is simply a release of surface tension, as opposed to a deeply experienced physical release that involves the whole body. This woman describes the difference very clearly.

Sometimes I feel an urgent need to come (usually on my own, when I haven't seen my lover for ages and haven't had much sex). When this happens I can come very quickly from touching myself but the actual orgasm is a bit of an anticlimax, as though I just need to release something. This is very different from the building passion that turns to divine tension inside me as I make love with my lover. There is a point at which I know I am going to come and often I like to spin that time out so that I am bursting for the release of orgasm. When my lover touches me or as I rub against her, I feel a combination of deepening, relaxing, and melting, and also tensing of my entire body as my heart and metabolism speed up. As I build towards an orgasm, I feel joyously frenzied. Sometimes it's a primal feeling like a wild animal and I like to grunt and make noise. As I come, I feel my insides melting and expanding, becoming alive. My whole body pulses. Often I find I quickly come again, maybe three times or so.

Pulsing and Contractions

The "pulsing" mentioned in the previous quote is fairly common. I've sometimes felt my lover pulsing at two- to four-second intervals for quite a long time (five minutes or more) after a strong orgasm. It may be localized in the vagina or in the genital area or it may be felt throughout the body, a little like very light muscle contractions. Pulsing may be an external indication of uterine contractions. It seems to be involuntary, and nothing like as strong as the tightening that occurs just prior to orgasm, or voluntary contraction of the PC muscles, which, when they are in good condition, can be very powerful. (Please refer to page 267 for more on the PC muscle.)

I occasionally feel and see a very active pulse that may involve my whole leg.

The pulsing reaches a crescendo and then fades, sometimes in thirty seconds, and sometimes over several minutes.

According to Masters and Johnson, the female orgasm involves a series of rhythmic muscular contractions (numbering from three to twelve) in the vagina. This gives rise to an image that is a little misleading, since rhythmic contractions cannot always be felt by the person who is doing the penetrating. The lesbians I spoke with say they are only occasionally able to feel rhythmic contractions in the vagina (apart from the pulsing mentioned earlier) when they are the doers. Most said they could feel a steady tightening around the entrance to the vagina leading up to the point of orgasm, and then a gradual relaxing afterwards. This steady contraction of the vaginal entrance may be so strong that it causes pain to the person doing the penetrating.

The reason rhythmic contractions aren't as obvious as we may think they would be, may be due to the fact that the doer is often moving her fingers inside while her partner is coming. It may also be that the receiver's leg and belly muscles, or perhaps her whole body, are spasming and clenching, which would make it difficult to distinguish what is going on in the vagina. Or it may simply be that the muscle contractions are not very noticeable.

A number of women (by no means all) report that when they have a strong orgasm they can feel a contraction in the midpoint of the groin, which would seem to indicate that it is in the uterus. Sometimes they can feel these contractions for a matter of minutes after an orgasm. They usually describe it as almost painful, a little like menstrual cramps, and several women say they are more likely to feel this when they are premenstrual or on their period. Afterwards they feel more relaxed in that area. Orgasms are known to relieve menstrual pain.

When I'm crampy from my period, I sometimes feel an orgasm in my uterus and it may be painful, but then when the contraction releases I feel better.

The external signs of orgasm can vary as much as the internal experience, and they may last for a few seconds or for hours. The same woman may react quite differently at different times. Sometimes she may thrash around and scream. Sometimes the whole body contracts or shakes and shudders. Her limbs may flutter, her feet and hands may stretch out and curl up. Her face may contort or it may remain quite serene. Sometimes she may hold quite still and be very quiet when she comes, merely arching or stretching the body a little. The intensity of the orgasm can't be measured by visible movement. Sometimes the most powerful ones are the ones that pass through deep inside, or on a level that is not physical, leaving few cues for an onlooker.

Pregnancy and Orgasm

It may initially seem surprising that some women feel more sexual when they are pregnant. But, after all, the uterus is part of a woman's sexual organs, and it changes continually as the fetus grows. The increase in size of the uterus may result in pressure on the G spot, resulting in spontaneous sexual arousal.

The only time I ever had an orgasm in my sleep was in the latter stages of pregnancy.

The contractions that occur during an orgasm may precipitate childbirth, and consequently women who are at risk for preterm labor are advised against sexual activity during pregnancy.

The medical establishment has tried to divorce the experience of giving birth from sexuality, and indeed many women cannot imagine it as anything but an exhausting, sterile, and pain-filled experience. However, some women do find themselves feeling sexually excited during the delivery process, and deliberate sexual arousal may greatly ease the experience.

A Vocabulary for Orgasm

If we lived in a society that communicated freely and openly about sex, there would have to be at least a dozen words to describe the different kinds of orgasm. The fact that there are only three (orgasm, coming, and climax) and that there are no standard definitions for the differences between them is an appalling indication of how little we comprehend the scope of sexual experience. Most of us grow up thinking there is some average kind of orgasmic experience, and that's what normal women have. What a limiting view, and a far cry from the truth!

The word **climax** is sometimes used to mean the latter part of the orgasm, or the peak. Some women use the word **coming** to mean the moment before release, the preparation to reaching the peak, prior to going over the edge into full orgasm. One woman described a feeling she calls coming that is different from orgasm:

It's a swelling, exploding feeling, but without the post-orgasmic body relaxation.

The experience of orgasm covers a huge range of intensity. It may involve the whole body, or it may be focused in certain parts of the body, or it may be an out-of-body experience. Why a woman has a particular experience one time and not another is often impossible to pin down because there are far too many variables: not just what is being done to her physically but her relationship to her partner, her surroundings, her state of mind, her emotional state, and everything that has led up to the moment of orgasm. One thing seems clear: any imposed classification used to define the phenomenon of female orgasm is not going to be useful, it is only going to be limiting. Fortunately, many of us are celebrating our diversity, instead of worrying that we aren't adhering to some artificial standard of "normality."

Multiple Orgasms

Most women (perhaps all) are capable of experiencing multiple orgasms, and many do so regularly. Some women don't care if they only have one, and others, like myself, don't feel satisfied if they have fewer than three.

My average orgasms are probably typical multiple orgasms. Each one lasts from three to maybe ten seconds, and I need a break of at least twenty seconds between each one, to let my clitoris get desensitized so I can take more stimulation. If the break is much longer than a minute I probably come too far down to get back up again. The second and the third are usually the strongest and they happen very quickly, with very little stimulation. The most I've ever had in one session was thirteen.

The length of the break between orgasms varies for different people, from a few seconds to a few minutes. Of course, if it's a few minutes you could describe it as a whole separate orgasm rather than one of a multiple. But women don't come down all the way out of a state of arousal in a few minutes, so it's really just a matter of how far down they need to come before they can take more stimulation to come back up. Most women can probably experience three or four orgasms during one lovemaking session. There seem to be a few women who don't, who are really and truly finished after that one big one.

I can't imagine having multiple orgasms. I can build up to another one after five minutes or so but the second one is never as satisfying.

Larger, longer orgasms tend to be multiple. Like when one orgasm continues like a skipped stone.

I am very likely to have an orgasm every time I have sex or masturbate. It's less a question of whether I have one, and more about how many and how intense.

I've always had multiple orgasms. I probably average three or four orgasms at one go. But if I make love all night, I can come constantly, and have different kinds of orgasm: from rubbing together with clothes on or without, from penetration with fingers or hand, from oral sex, or from my body being stroked in just the right way.

Once I came thirty-two times. After a while my boyfriend just sat back amazed, and watched me stimulate myself for the last ten or so orgasms.

In the next chapter we'll look at how different women experience the flows of energy in their bodies when they come. To close this chapter, here are a few words from Joy on defining an orgasm:

I have a vast variety of orgasms. I see stars, rockets, and all kinds of other visuals. Some feel like jumping out of a plane. Or they're like an ocean swell, and sometimes the surf is so strong it sweeps me away; other times it just laps at the shore. They can be very deep, where all my internal organs go into pleasant spasm; maybe my knees go weak, suddenly all the tension drains down and out of my body. Sometimes they are like earthquakes, but more commonly they're like waves. They're often electrical: I feel the electrical energy moving up and down central channels inside my body, not on the surface. They can be either vaginally or clitorally centered. But when they're clitorally centered, it's like that three centimeters of flesh is the whole universe.

4
CHAPTER

The Energetic Experience of Orgasm

My orgasms are exquisite and deep, like riding a wave, exciting, wild, raw energy, primal, deeply satisfying. The buildup is a warm, flowing, pleasantly exciting sensation that keeps building to more excitement. It's fun to hang out there for a while. Orgasm brings the excitement to a peak that satisfies a deep body longing and leaves me glowing, ecstatic, and floating. It's a feeling of being deeply bonded with the universe.

There's a building of intensity of feeling, I feel like I'm becoming pure energy, ceasing to be a clearly defined physical body with boundaries. It's like I can clearly perceive being an energetic being of vibrating molecules, part of and one with the woman I'm with and everything in the universe. I experience this in differing degrees of intensity depending on my situation. Then orgasm itself is like a wave of energy cresting inside me and through me, a release of the buildup of energy within me, truly ecstatic and totally exquisite. This is also accompanied by my muscles contracting and shuddering, often very strongly — yes, the earth does move for me!

Sexuality can put us in touch with powerful flows of energy that we may not otherwise have a reason or the ability to access. Thinking of orgasm in terms of energy flow can be very useful, enabling us to visualize it in a much broader way than the merely physical. The same is true of life; understanding it as occurring on a plane of energy allows us to comprehend some of the unseen forces that affect us.

Orgasm is about highly focused energy, and being orgasmic is about learning to let our bodies focus energy while we let go of trying to control it. This may seem like a paradox: surely if you are focusing energy, then you are controlling it. But there is a big difference between controlling a flow of energy — trying to force it to move in a particular pattern — and removing blocks that are preventing a natural flow so that we can allow our bodies to do what they want to do: gather, focus, and release the energy.

Cultural conditioning teaches us to block this natural flow. When we overcome our conditioning and allow ourselves to be freely carried by the energy that is released during orgasm, then we release the potential to have transcendental experiences. Sexual energy is very powerful: it is, after all, the energy that creates and sustains life.

It is perfectly possible to learn to channel the flow of energy during orgasm. Various methods have been developed for doing this. Most of these methods include experiencing high levels of sexual ecstasy. Some of them are discussed at the end of this chapter and in Chapter Five.

The Nonphysical Components of Orgasm

It has been said that the brain is the most important sex

organ. In reality, I believe the factors that turn us on are often beyond the comprehension of the logical brain, such as smell, sound, long forgotten memories, and inexplicable energies that we aren't consciously aware of. Sexual arousal in dreams epitomizes this phenomenon. A number of women have had the experience of waking up out of an erotic dream in a high state of arousal, yet without any of the normal signs: no throbbing clitoris, no wet and swollen lips. It is as though the excitement occurs on an ethereal level, where we are not actually *in* the body we normally inhabit.

Paradoxically, sex is based in the physical and yet it may take us beyond the physical. Many women report feeling overwhelmed and transported by orgasm, and what they seem to mean is that a powerful sense of contained energy builds inside their bodies and then releases. The energy can manifest visually, aurally, physically, emotionally, spiritually. Physical stimulation, although certainly important, is only one contributing factor; our best and strongest orgasms seem to be the ones that involve us on other levels as well as the physical. These other levels have been variously labeled mental, intellectual, emotional, spiritual, psychological, psychic, and chemical (as in having great "chemistry" with someone). Because all of the experiences described by these words are extremely subjective, we have no consensus definitions of what they actually mean.

In this and the following chapter, I shall attempt to illustrate what these words and phrases mean to different people, and what place they have in sexual arousal. Some women equate the mental with the spiritual, since they find that once they are able to quiet their minds they enter a stillness that is an experience of oneness. Other women equate the spiritual with the emotional, and have their best orgasms when they feel a heart connection with their partner. Some people might not differentiate between emotional, psychic, and spiritual ecstasy.

An orgasm can be triggered by an overwhelming sense of joy or love, perhaps from the connection with a partner, or just from experiencing intense pleasure or beauty. The natural beauty of the environment can add a whole different dimension to a sexual experience:

My best orgasm ever was when I was sleeping out on a deck with my lover, and we woke up just before dawn and started to make love. Then a flock of yellow birds flew down towards us, and we both came together just as the first of the sun's rays touched us. I felt out of my skin.

The inspiration for an orgasm need not come from physical stimulation, and there may be little or no buildup. Some women come in their sleep, from a powerful dream; or they are able to generate a flow of sexual energy by using fantasy or mental focus, with some muscle control. Jana talks about orgasms that creep up on her almost against her will. She is a Buddhist monk, in the habit of sitting in meditation for very long periods of time. She's not the asexual person you might imagine a monk to be; she masturbates once or twice a day. Sometimes as she sits in meditation she finds an orgasm coming over her without any conscious intention on her part:

The feeling runs away by itself and my mind focuses in on itself and I'm going, "Oh my god oh my god oh my god ...." I'm sitting there having an orgasm, hoping no one notices. It's amazing how strong the feeling gets.

Laura had her first ever orgasm watching a horse race; no one was touching her, nor was she touching herself, and she wasn't even thinking about sex:

The beauty and vitality and competitive spirit of the horses just took me to orgasm!

It is not unusual for an intensely pleasurable experience to find an outlet in orgasm even though it is not (at least initially) a specifically sexual pleasure.

One night I was lying on my bed with the window open. It was warm, and a delightful sensuous breeze was wafting over me. I opened my legs to it and felt as if it was actually caressing me. I stayed with the feeling until I came.

I've had an orgasm a few times listening to very intense, passionate music.

One woman reported that when she was getting a massage, not being touched in her genital area, and unaware of any sexual arousal, she suddenly found herself coming. Dee reports finding her body shaken by an orgasm as she sat on a rock by a river watching her lover walk along the shore. Apparently, deep feelings of love or joy or enthusiasm can unexpectedly give rise to exactly the same physiological response as physical stimulation, and can be experienced as an ecstatic energy release.

A number of women report that they can come from

imagining sex, without any external stimulus, which is a little different from having an orgasm come unexpectedly out of thin air.

On occasion I've been able to come just from visualizing sensual intercourse, without anyone touching me, or me touching myself.

I have had an orgasm from a purely mental fantasy about someone, without touching myself or having anyone touch me.

When I've had the experience of orgasm without any stimulation, it was like a flashback and a brief shiver all over and a tingle to my clit. It doesn't matter what I'm doing. I could be lying down, driving a car, relaxing, whatever.

Sometimes the only external stimulus that's necessary is another person's voice.

I've rarely had an orgasm without any stimulation at all but it has happened when I've been on the phone to my lover.

I can have a vaginal orgasm very easily, just from being told to come, if I've been having a lot of sex over a number of days.

The "telling" can be verbal or otherwise: her lover might be across the room at the time. One woman said that she could come simply from seeing her lover make suggestive finger movements. An emotional component — a strong current of love between partners — may be present in some of these cases, but it certainly isn't necessary for all women who experience this kind of orgasm. It may occur in part because the woman is in a state of sexual excitement already. Many women find it possible to remain in a highly aroused state for a long time without experiencing discomfort.

I can go through my day feeling constantly aroused. I'll be walking down the street and the feeling deep down in my groin gets more and more intense, just from the motion of walking, especially if I'm wearing jeans, and I find myself coming. I have to stop and lean against a wall.

Because phone sex and on-line sex often occur between people who don't know each other well, or even at all, we can assume there is no emotional connection. This kind of sex uses the power of words to create physical sensations. For some women, the words create erotic visual images, and thus work just like a fantasy. For others, the sound and the meaning of the words bypass the mental realm altogether and go straight into physical sensations. When two people are physically present, a glance, body language, a facial expression, or simply a casually stated innuendo can all have similar effects. A very strong feeling of love can produce erotic sensations without any physical stimulation, and vice versa: erotic physical or mental stimulation can produce intense feelings of love. The physical, the mental, and the emotional become one. They are all erotic sensations: you have a feeling of love for someone and it gives rise to a mental picture that is erotic and therefore creates a physical response; someone touches you in a nonsexual way and you feel flooded with love for that person, and you are suddenly aware of your pelvic muscles contracting; and so on, the permutations are endless. And they can all give rise to a sense of oneness that, for some, may have spiritual significance.

Chemistry: A Psychic Connection

I have an occasional lover who brings me to orgasm in a way no one else ever has. He is an accomplished lover, and my attraction to him as a person is so chemically/spiritually/obsessively intense that I can't tell what influences what.

Many of us have experienced an energy flow between ourselves and another person that is not of our conscious creation at all: we call it **attraction**, or in its most extreme forms, **falling in love**. It can be anything from a mild sexual response, to overwhelming body chemistry, to divine mania. **Chemistry** is a confusing term here; the attraction may be chemical — that is, caused by pheromones that stimulate us on a subconscious level — but it may also be interpreted as an attraction that occurs on a psychic level. Whether you call it psychic or chemical, it is a flow of energy. It's feasible to learn how to play with this energy, consciously making it greater or smaller, bringing it to an orgasmic release, or not. What is important, as with all sexual play, is that it be consensual. Perhaps one of the people involved is taking it much more seriously than the other(s). Check this out before you get carried away with it.

Strong attraction is not necessarily about an emotional connection, but for many women the two are synonymous. A strong emotional component, or heart connection, with another person certainly has the power to bring on an orgasm, sometimes as much as anything physical. These two women were awed and amazed by the spontaneous orgasms that occurred with particular men:

We were just lying together in bed, and I felt this pure ecstasy filling my body; pure spirit. I trembled and my body glowed, my groin became bathed in warmth and sensation, which lasted several minutes, and then I orgasmed.

I was so in love with a man once that my orgasm, which usually follows all the stages of arousal, plateau, orgasm, resolution, etc., just came out of nowhere so quickly I felt transported.

Some women really seem to need to experience a heart connection in order to allow sexual energy to flow between themselves and their lover, while others don't. Women who have multiple partners are judged harshly by our society; there is a widespread assumption that we cannot experience a heart connection with someone whom we don't know well, or haven't made a lifelong commitment to. I think this is a misconception: I believe it *is* possible to have a very deep connection with someone you have just met, simply because you resonate with that person, because there is some kind of connection on a psychic level. And it is certainly possible to feel very strongly for more than one person at a time. Our language fails to supply nondisparaging words to describe these relationships. What seems to be true is that some women cannot be open on a heart level until they know their partner well, and other women can be very open on a heart level when they first meet someone.

The mental and emotional components are important. I must feel trust. But sometimes it's easier with someone I don't know — they haven't betrayed me yet, they're fresh.

The emotions that are brought into play by an intense attraction are an essential aspect of arousal for some women. Jesse calls this the "romantic element." For her, good sex must include romance. She must feel a strong attraction for her sexual partner. Joy is quite the opposite. For her, sex is about having fun, and she can even sleep with someone she doesn't particularly like, and have very good sex with plenty of orgasms. I am very picky about my close friends, but if the chemistry (or the psychic/emotional connection, or whatever you want to call it) is right, I can enjoy an affair with someone I don't particularly want to spend a lot of time with out of bed. With such a person, I will make sure not to make any emotional commitments; I don't want any pretense about what we are sharing or not sharing.

While orgasm is not necessarily an emotional experience for all women, very few women seem to be able to come with their partner when they are holding negative emotions towards that person. A number of women described the buildup of negative emotion within a relationship, and then withholding those emotions in a sexual context, making it harder for them to let go into orgasm. Victoria stopped having orgasms after the first year of her first long-term relationship and for a long time she thought there was something wrong with her. After she left her lover, she realized that she had closed down emotionally, and that was why she had ceased to have orgasms.

Emotional Orgasms

Many women find that the best sex arises out of an emotional connection, and for some, feeling loved and appreciated by their partner is essential.

My orgasms seem to depend on the emotional state that is created between my partner and myself (other than masturbation, which is always a successful release). When I feel cared for, when his attention is fully with me, when he seems interested in who I am as a person and what and how I feel, then I can open my heart freely, and only then can I open my body freely, and allow orgasm.

The experience of orgasm itself can bring up a lot of emotion. Jesse clearly labeled an emotional orgasm:

Sometimes my heart breaks open and melts. It doesn't come from my genitals, but otherwise it's an awful lot like an orgasm.

Donna described having orgasms that felt "difficult" emotionally, orgasms that revealed more of her vulnerability than she was comfortable with. Sometimes she even consciously put a stop to them. I am sure that many women learn to put stops on their orgasms either consciously or unconsciously, precisely because they don't want to be emotionally exposed.

I have certainly had the experience of an orgasm that was almost more of an emotional release than a physical one. Usually when this occurs, I am aware that I need an emotional release, but sometimes that awareness prevents me from feeling free to be sexual in the first place. Sex often feels too dangerous when I'm in a very vulnerable space.

Tears are also not uncommon for women when they come.

Sometimes there is an explosion that seems to reach other dimensions and often leaves me weeping in a state of exquisite longing for that other dimension. It is as if my whole life were a plea to live in that place and the tears are of gratitude for touching that place, and for sadness that it seems so rare.

Making love is very emotional for me. If things aren't going well in my heart, even if I think they are, my orgasm releases a huge well of sadness within me and I cry and cry and cry, mostly just streaming tears, no sobs.

It seems as though the physical release triggers an emotional release that has been waiting for an outlet.

Often after an orgasm I will feel very sad, and the feeling builds until I cry and cry and cry. I don't mind it; in fact, I feel very good after the storm is over. Sometimes I'm amazed at the depth of the sadness and sobbing. I think I get a load of sadness from just being in the world and seeing and hearing about so many sad, horrible, unjust events that my body just wants to release it periodically, and it uses the orgasm as a trigger.

One woman complained that her partners don't want to know what she's feeling at these times.

The thing that gets me is guys never ask why I'm crying! I guess they're afraid to know.

Sometimes the experience of being flooded with grief or emotional pain comes instead of, rather than accompanying an orgasm, especially if a woman is having trouble coming. It may be that the tears provide the necessary release, in lieu of a physical climax.

Sometimes I feel like I really need to come and I just can't get there. When this happens I nearly always end up crying.

Sometimes if I'm making love and I don't have an orgasm, I get completely out of control emotionally and burst into floods of tears.

But the emotion an orgasm triggers may just as easily be joy, with laughter as part of the orgasmic release. And some women find that having an orgasm calms them down and relaxes them when they are feeling emotional.

When I'm feeling sad or lonely, I sometimes comfort myself by masturbating to orgasm. My relationship to myself and the sense of being in control of my body feels really good.

The Intellectual Component: Focusing the Mind

Some women feel that conscious intention is an essential ingredient to orgasm. Marya says that she has to make a mental decision to climax, as though giving herself permission before it can happen. Although most of the women I interviewed said there was *not* an intellectual aspect to coming, quite a few reported that they were more likely to have orgasms if they felt their partner was in control on the mental plane, or was an intellectually stimulating person. This might manifest as someone who is verbal during sexual play, or in other words, someone with good patter!

I love it when my lover talks dirty to me and fantasizes verbally.

In reality, there may be much more of an intellectual component to orgasm than we think. Perhaps it would be more accurate to say that one of the ways we block ourselves from orgasm is with the power of our conscious minds, because of an emotionally-based intellectual belief that it is not okay to let go. This is borne out by one woman who, for a long time, only came in her sleep. Her waking mind could not allow her to let go enough. We can develop an intellectual belief, which we then exert through the will, as a result of something that holds a big emotional charge. I don't think it's possible to delineate clear boundaries between the emotional and the intellectual. Our bodies can be affected by emotional or physical trauma in such a way that they respond without any *conscious* brain involvement. Since we have a strong tendency to want to rationalize our behavior, there is often no way for us to know when a physical response is due to a body memory of a trauma that has been forgotten by the conscious mind, rather than a rationale-based conclusion. It can be very hard to see when the emotional becomes intellectualized. Moreover, we tend to want to hold onto our rational beliefs, and we may get upset when they are challenged. Then the intellectual becomes emotional.

Most of us are brought up to value the intellectual and denigrate the emotional. Yet the truth is, we are far more swayed by our feelings than we like to admit: we make the pretense of being rational by trying to overlay our feelings with rational explanations. Our feelings never lie, but our intellects are affected by "oughts" and "shoulds." Thus our minds try to make us fit into the status quo, even when it is not right for us.

Some women can "think" themselves into orgasm, with-out stimulation from any source other than their own minds. This usually means focusing very intently on a fantasy, but sometimes what happens is not so specific, and it certainly need not include imagery of genital stimulation. We don't really have the words to describe what it is, but it's something like "thinking oneself into the feeling of orgasm."

I use my mind. I let go. I want it, so it happens. It's simple for me. There is nothing more to tell.

In her book, *Women Who Love Sex* (Pocket Books, 1994), Gina Ogden has a whole chapter devoted to "thinking off." She took one of her subjects into a lab and measured for all the signs of orgasm as the woman came without touching herself and barely moving. The measurements were exactly what you would expect for an orgasm brought on by any physical method: high heart rate and blood pressure, dilated pupils, reduced sensitivity to pain, and heightened sensual responses.

Many women fantasize when they are masturbating or when they are with a partner, and the fantasy may really help them to get off. Some women read erotica or watch movies or look at pictures. Fantasizing is an intellectual skill: it requires an active mind, a vivid imagination, and the ability to concentrate. Joy has had orgasms while she was writing, apparently just from the intellectual thrill.

A couple of times I have come from a psychological turn-on, when I'm off in my head and there's no physical stimulation. It's connected to the excitement of creativity, usually when I'm writing something that has an erotic charge for me. It might be something that someone else would not find erotic at all.

Learning to focus the mind can have remarkable results, as anyone who has meditated over a long period will tell you. Freud's idea that the sensation of orgasm should migrate from the clitoris to the vagina may actually be accomplished by someone who chooses to think the sensation there, but one can also think the sensation to anywhere else on the body (fingers, earlobes, different chakras, wherever). People with spinal cord injuries, who have no sensation in their genital area, can still experience sexual feelings, and may have very satisfying sexual relationships.

Some women say they cannot come if their brains are going a mile a minute, while others are able to keep their brains occupied with a fantasy. A few women do not come without a fantasy to help them focus, and this often involves images of being raped. Generally, such fantasies are about giving themselves permission to relinquish control; the conscious brain won't let go until it is tricked into thinking that someone else is forcing it to do so!

Personally, I often find there is part of my brain that tends to isolate itself from the rest of me when I am having an orgasm. While my body is in the throes of intense convulsions, my brain might be busy thinking about the color of the walls. As long as it's not a thought that makes me anxious, I can usually let it go so that it doesn't interfere with my pleasure, but I have more intense and longer orgasms when I totally switch my brain off. I think my brain's desire to absent itself during sex is a leftover from my childhood sexual experiences.

Aftershocks

My experience with purely mental or emotional stimulation is that it can be very exciting, but often in a rather diffuse sense. If it is very genitally focused, which it might be if I am reading or looking at erotica, I'm not usually able to bring the energy to release without touching myself or moving around. Occasionally, when I've been sitting still concentrating on writing or some other creative outlet, I have a kind of upper body shudder that is definitely a release of energy and might be considered a kind of orgasm. I have also had experiences along the lines of what Jesse describes here:

Sometimes when I'm very turned on, I get single contractions that feel just like aftershock contractions, and recently I had a short set of these from an intense and intimate turn-on with almost no touching of any kind, just prolonged eye contact, and then a slow movement towards each other that culminated in my lover brushing the side of her face against mine. I believe now that this might be considered an orgasm, but I hadn't thought of it as such because there wasn't the usual physical buildup leading to it.

The aftershock contractions that Jesse refers to are something many women experience: they are like little jolts that jerk your body around, and they may occur after particularly intense sex. Terry describes having aftershocks, "like little orgasms," for days. In a similar vein, a number of women report a powerful sinking feeling in their gut when they think about an exceptional sexual experience:

Sometimes I'll be walking along daydreaming about having sex and all of a sudden that feeling comes over me, and my guts jolt. It's often accompanied by an involuntary moan that is obviously sexual, and that's very embarrassing if someone else is around!

The day after exciting sex, part of me sometimes stays turned on, and even doing mundane things, my mind suddenly flashes to what we did the night before and I'll get a little momentary orgasm that makes me jump or shudder.

Simultaneous and Empathic Orgasms

Simultaneous orgasm is the ultimate goal for many people. Like any goal, it can set us up for a sense of failure, since it is often difficult to achieve. A few lucky people are inspired to come at the same moment as their lover. It seems to be a glorious feat, to be so in tune with your partner that your energy is carried into orgasm with his or hers. I have had a few lovers who were brought to orgasm by my coming, but I've never achieved it the other way round. A couple of men commented that they were brought to orgasm by their partners:

After she has her first orgasm from manual stimulation I will sometimes move to penile insertion, and in most instances reach simultaneous orgasm with her second one.

One man had this to say about how wonderful it was:

On the one and only time to date that we have had simultaneous orgasm through intercourse, it was simply indescribable, out of this world, fantastic!!!

A number of women referred to a kind of orgasm that I have called "empathic." These might be simultaneous or they might not. They occur when a woman is making love to someone else, and she gets so excited by her lover's response — by his or her arousal — that she finds herself coming. It is the energy of her lover's turn-on that creates her orgasm. Some women experience it as an unexpected bonus, something that just comes out of the blue: their body goes into automatic orgasm, with no awareness of any buildup, no conscious desire to come, no conscious seeking of orgasm.

It's always a surprise because I'm never expecting it.

Lesbians who experience this phenomenon stress that it was a very different kind of orgasm from the kind they have when partners are making love to each other simultaneously.

I find it distracting if someone is making love to me at the same time as I'm making love to her. I can't concentrate on what I'm doing to my lover. However, the kind of turn-on I feel through me making love to someone else is not a distraction.

The kind of orgasm that I am calling empathic occurs purely as a result of what a woman is doing to someone else; it is part and parcel of what she is doing to that person, it enhances what she is doing, and it doesn't distract at all. Her awareness is all on her partner; there is no direct stimulation of her own genitals. And her orgasm may well occur simultaneously with her partner's.

There have been a dozen or so times when I've come from making love to my partner, without being touched myself. I think there is a sort of psychic/sexual connection in which boundaries melt and fuse.

In heterosexual sex, the emphasis is very often on what

the man is doing to the woman; he is usually the one dictating the action, and he is often focusing on gearing up to the moment of intercourse. In this scenario, there may not necessarily be much opportunity for the woman to focus on pleasuring him, although it doesn't have to be like this, as Donna illustrates:

I almost always come from making love to my partner, especially when I'm sucking his penis. I find the rhythm extremely exciting and the sensation of sucking invites my hips to move and my uterus to contract. It's also very exciting to feel his excitement mounting and the contractions I can feel in him before he reaches orgasm.

Energy Movement Within the Body

Some women are more aware than others of the flow of energy in and through their physical bodies during sexual play. Linci has worked with this as part of her spiritual practice. When she describes making love to another woman, she says that the energy moves in circles between her and her lover, from one woman's chakras to the other and back, around and around. But the actual orgasm, if it's not an empathic one, produces energy that moves vertically in a linear path, either up or down her body.

Jana finds that the energy of orgasm moves differently if she has been deep in meditation:

Instead of building up and exploding outwards like a beautiful flower, it builds through my body more slowly and then moves out sideways. Everything goes into quietude without exploding first.

Most women agreed that the energy gathers in the pelvic area and then goes up, down, or directly outwards from there. For Donna, the energy gathers in her upper body if she's having her nipples stimulated (she can come from nipple stimulation alone). Whatever brings the orgasm on, once it is under way, she says the energy moves upwards vertically from her body, into her lover if he's lying on top of her.

Many women say they find themselves stretching their feet out when they come, as though to let the energy flow out their soles.

I have to have my legs straight out, and I can't bear to have limited space for my feet.

Jean normally experiences the energy moving directly out of her feet, but she had a one-time experience that is very interesting:

My partner had her hand over my throat as I was coming, restricting my breathing. The energy shot up to the top of my head and then bounced back down and shot out of my feet, leaving my legs weak and shaky, like all the nerve endings had been fired off. It was amazing!

Since limiting the oxygen to the brain can have the effect of increasing the level of arousal and enhancing orgasms, the practice of breathing restriction is not uncommon. The problem with this is that it can also kill you, and it can do so extremely fast — much faster than you might realize. If you decide to play around with this, *be very careful.* Don't take it to an extreme, and do it only with people you trust to be one hundred percent attentive to you. **Never allow anything** around your throat or over your mouth that cannot be removed in an instant; never put anything over your mouth that might be inhaled.

The experience most commonly reported seems to be that the energy moves down the legs and out through the feet, and sometimes out through the hands as well. Some women feel it going up and out of their heads, which is likely to be accompanied by a feeling of oneness with the universe. This most often occurs when there is a strong emotional bond between lovers, following a lot of sexual play. A sense of spaciness, and a sense of oneness, may occur when the higher chakras have been opened up, and an orgasm is certainly capable of doing this. The energy of orgasm may even carry us to another realm of consciousness. Many women report that they have had the sensation of floating after orgasm, and they experience themselves as something other than physical.

Waves of pleasure build into towering walls of energy that wash over and lift and toss me about, and I cry out like a flock of birds. I don't feel confined to my body. I lose my physical edges. Post-orgasm, I feel very warm and glowing, although my body sometimes aches for a few days after.

Once I had a total out-of-body experience. I was up there hovering a few inches above myself, watching myself have an orgasm.

Alignment

The physical position of the body can often affect a woman's ability to have an orgasm or, at least, to have a strong orgasm. It may be important to notice what position your body is choosing as it approaches orgasm.

I went through a period when I felt compelled to cross my legs even though it meant I wouldn't have such a satisfying orgasm; it was as if I needed to limit the physical intensity. I don't know why.

I feel that I must physically align my body to allow the movement of energy. I find I can only come with my whole body stretched out and arched; all my muscles tense up harder and harder as I get closer to coming. It's as though my body requires it in order for the energy to be able to release. I tend to hold my breath as I approach the orgasm (or it approaches me), but the actual release often necessitates me making a sound, a kind of a groan, or perhaps words, so then I take deep breaths. And breathing into my belly makes the orgasm happen. The energy that has gathered pours outwards, mostly flooding down my legs and out of my feet. I am often aware of my feet feeling electric, and my legs shaking afterwards. Sometimes I feel the energy in my throat.

Because of the way I come, I always do so lying on my back, where I or my partner has plenty of space to manipulate my clitoris in the necessary manner. Many women say they like to have their legs straight, although it doesn't matter to everyone. Jean also stretches herself out; however, unlike me, she is able to come lying on her front. She arches her back in the same way, but uses a vibrator on the bed against her clitoris, so that the arching of her body pushes her pelvis into the bed, and her clitoris harder against the vibrator.

There are plenty of women who can come in a number of different positions, including standing up.

I love having sex standing up. Lying down dissipates the energy. I think I'm trained to come standing up because when I was a kid I did it a lot in the shower.

My orgasms are more exciting when I'm lying on my back with my legs drawn up. Being on all fours or prone slows it down.

I notice that orgasm feels very different in different positions: I can differentiate between those experienced on my back, on my front, and standing up.

Visuals

The energy of an orgasm may create colors or scenery in the mind's eye. Donna and Terry both see patterns of flashing lights, constellations of stars connected with lines.

I see lots of yellow and white, some red and orange. They're mostly hot, bright colors, not black. I see starbursts and sunbursts of different colors. One is a deep brilliant blue. I experience it in my third eye and it feels wonderful. I can hang out there on that plateau before orgasm with that deep blue, for a long time.

Joy has some fascinating visuals, from psychedelic light shows to more mundane and often strange visuals, such as nuts and bolts rolling down a hill, weird animals, odd postcard collections, or bizarre, not necessarily idyllic, landscapes. When she and her lover have simultaneous orgasms, they may see the same images. On one occasion they both had a sensation of hopping, and saw rabbits popping up out of holes. It was, Joy said, a very friendly, cheerful lovemaking session!

According to Lisa, the energy of the sex affects the colors she sees:

If it's a lovemaking experience, then I might see really soft earth colors, corals, and watery colors, flowing blues and aquas. I get the same kind of visuals when I'm giving someone a massage. If it's bad-ass sex, nasty sex, then I see black. I see leather.

When Lisa talks about "bad-ass" sex, she doesn't mean that it isn't a wonderful consensual experience, she just means her desire has a different flavor — she is not feeling sweet and gentle. This brings up a very interesting point, that the energy we bring to sexual play can vary considerably on different occasions. I discuss this in detail in Chapter Nine.

The Power of Fantasy

Jesse is another woman who relates to the concept of energy flows and she is also someone who finds fetish and fantasy a wonderful source of orgasms. She describes something that might be called an imaginary orgasm that shoots from an imaginary penis. Jesse has no desire to be a man, but she plays around with fantasies of being a man in bed. She can come in a number of different ways, including when she has a dildo strapped on and is having "intercourse" in the missionary position with her female lover. The energy of these shooting orgasms moves in an outwardly direction. Some women say that an orgasm from using a strapped-on dildo happens because the base of the dildo presses on the clitoris, or on the G spot from the outside. But it is also possible that the psychological element of fantasy is a major factor in such an orgasm. Jesse's shooting orgasms can also occur when *she* is being penetrated, if she is fantasizing that she has a male anatomy.

Jean reports a similar shooting sensation, when some part of her is being sucked on (toes, fingers, or dildo — yes, she does think of the dildo as part of her, when she's wearing it) and says that when she comes like this, she feels as though she has a penis. The energy is a rushing feeling through her body, an "outward explosion," but the climax is not as satisfying as other kinds because it leaves her with some tension.

One of the questionnaire respondents said she had experienced this, but only with one lover:

I once had a lover who inspired me to come when she came. It felt like a very male type of orgasm, like I had a penis and was coming from out of it.

When two people get together, the combination of their energies may create quite a different experience from anything either of them have had before. This can be frustrating when you get together with someone new and the same activities don't feel quite as good as they did with the last person. But if you are willing to experiment in new ways with new lovers, it can also be exciting, and at least you know that every experience is unique. Sex never has to be routine.

Sound

Many women talk about a connection between the throat and the pelvic area. Interestingly, if you examine a diagram of the throat and a diagram of the female sexual organs, you will see that they look similar. According to Hindu tradition, there is a direct link between the second chakra, which is the center of sex and emotion, based three fingers below the belly button, and the fifth chakra, located in the throat, which relates to self-expression and making sounds. Moving the energy in the one area will tend to affect the other area. This is borne out by a number of women:

There is a shift in my throat when I'm close to coming, like the feeling I get when I begin to sing. There's definitely some subtle correlation between my throat and my genital area. I have to allow the muscles in my throat to soften so that my breath can move more freely. Any sound I make will often carry the orgasm for a longer period of time than if I am silent.

Yelling out really helps to release the energy of orgasm for me. I'm a very noisy lovemaker and that's an important part of sexual expression for me. If I have to be quiet I feel very constrained.

In her work as a tantric teacher, Jwala encourages women to use sound:

The throat chakra is the one that women really hold closed, holding in our expressions of anger and rage over the abuse we've suffered from centuries of patriarchy. I have women make noises even when they don't feel like it, to release stuck feelings and verbalize their rage. They can verbalize the act of pushing the abuser(s) out of their space.

I have found that opening my mouth and making a noise can sometimes carry me into orgasm, as though releasing the sound releases the energy of the orgasm. As Jwala says, because we often block the flow of energy through our bodies without being aware we are doing so, it is necessary to make a conscious decision to vocalize our passion, even though (or because) it feels uncomfortable.

Extended Orgasm

Many men and some women have an attitude toward sex that I call the get-it-over-with syndrome. They have a finite view of sex as a strictly functional act with orgasm at the end of it. When we can move beyond this limited view and accept a concept of sex as an enjoyable activity in itself without a beginning or an end, our possibilities are immediately expanded. But even when we relate to sex in that broader sense, we may still relate to orgasm as a finite experience, not expected to last more than a few seconds.

Extended sexual orgasm is a phrase generally used to refer to a sensation of orgasm that can last from a few minutes to six hours or more, in women and men. Depending on the person who is using the phrase, it can mean any one of the following:

- staying on the verge of orgasm, in a high state of arousal, just at the peak without going over;
- going over, and then staying in an actual prolonged physically orgasmic state;
- staying in the dreamlike state of oneness that may occur with orgasm, but without the attendant physical symptoms (body contractions and so on). This might also be described as the **afterglow**.

These are all very subjective experiences, and therefore difficult to clearly differentiate. It's highly unlikely for anyone to get to these states of arousal on a regular basis without skillful manual or oral stimulation of the clitoris and the G spot. But the physical aspects of stimulation, although important, are only about one quarter to one third of what causes these experiences to occur. Other important factors are communication with your partner, your partner's ability to read your body language, and your emotional and mental state: how much are you willing and able to give up your normal hold on reality in order to let yourself remain in such a state of bliss? Many of us have difficulty allowing ourselves to experience ecstasy for very long. We are not usually brought up to believe that pleasure in itself is a worthy goal. We are often more concerned about remaining "functional." There is a prevailing attitude that can be summed up as "get-it-over-with-and-get-on-with-life." The intensity and sense of "otherness" that comes with strong sexual feelings, pleasant though these may be for a few moments, can quickly become uncomfortable. It takes practice and motivation to stay with the sensations. But, as Jwala says, it is a skill that can be learned, and the benefits are remarkable:

We can learn to tolerate stronger sexual energy so that we don't block it off at the lower chakras, but allow it up to higher levels; if we can really bring it up to the top of the head and let it flow out of the seventh chakra, that is spiritual bliss, and we can be in an altered state for hours.

If you are withholding emotions from your partner, or your mind refuses to be still, or you are in a hurry, or you have issues about sex that prevent you from being fully present, you won't be able to stay in a prolonged orgasmic state. You need to trust your partner completely, and let go of *all* distractions, so that you can really relax. It has happened for me when I have a very strong heart connection, when I'm deeply in love and utterly focused. Then I find myself on an elevated plane of orgasm for a very long time without ever really seeming to come down: either nailed to the bed, or floating above it.

In her video, *The Sluts and Goddesses* (which I highly recommend, both for fun and for educational purposes!), Annie Sprinkle is on camera having an orgasm that lasts more than five minutes. There is a fine line between one continual orgasm and multiple orgasms that occur so closely together they can barely be distinguished. If extended orgasm was a commonly known phrase, I think a lot of the women who wrote the following would be using it to describe what is going on for them, instead of the better known phrase "multiple orgasm":

When I have multiple orgasms, it's like I've achieved a melding of the spirit. I've submitted, and I can stay at that elevated plane for a long time.

I have multiple orgasms and after the third or fourth one, they become a way of experiencing myself in vastness. They are something else, something very non-local. There's a lot of fluidity back and forth. I can make love for hours and come and come and come like that.

In her video, *Extended Sexual Orgasm for Men and Women,* Kathryn Grosz describes ESO as a heightened state of arousal, which she calls orgasm, with a climax at the end of it. The level of arousal may be greater than you normally reach before going over, but the climax itself is a separate event that signals the end of the extended part. She describes at length how to maintain this state of arousal: the doer gets the receiver up to as high a point as possible without actually going over, and then backs off or changes stimulation for a moment or two, before picking up the rhythm again. So the receiver is always "reaching out" for the sensation again, and each time she reaches out she moves up a little higher on the arousal scale. This can go on for an hour or more. The doer must change the speed or the type of stroke or pause for a second, in order to sustain the experience of peaking that occurs just before climax, and she or he has to divine when these pauses or changes are necessary by observing the body language of the receiver very closely.

This video shows two couples, a male/female, and a female/female. I was disappointed that the female/female couple weren't more physically passionate, and no identifiable female climax was shown, but apart from that, it is an educational and enjoyable film.

Alan and Donna Brauer are the authors of a book called *Extended Sexual Orgasm* (ESO) published by Warner Books. They clearly describe the kinds of muscular contractions that characterize ESO. They define it as a continuous, very intense experience of orgasm, that is reached after moving through one or more "normal" orgasms. Apart from this, there doesn't seem to be a substantial difference between their concept of ESO and Kathryn Grosz's. Their method of getting there seems to be very similar. It primarily involves switching the types of stimulation, from the G spot to the glans of the clitoris and back again, just at the point of orgasm, and repeating that sequence so that the sensation continues to build. They also discuss "reaching out" for the sensation.

Patricia Hunter is one of a team of three people who teaches these kinds of techniques to couples in the San Francisco Bay Area.

It's very important to learn to relax and let your body vibrate. I see it as one quarter of each of the following: mental, emotional, spiritual, and physical. You're never going to get off the ground with just the physical. I see the spiritual and the intuitive as being the same. If you're able to do the physical, the mental, and the intuitive, then that will take care of blocked emotions. But you have to stop being goal-oriented, and you must have communication skills. Good communication requires trust, surrender, and being able to read one another. ESO is holographic with the rest of life: you must confront life, and your fears, and go through the obstacles that your mind presents; you must have more of a will to pleasure than to pain. Tantric teachers are teaching sexuality and sensuality, which is part of the picture, but it's the difference between a dance party and being a champion ballroom dancer.

It's like boiling water; once you've reached that state of boiling you can stay there as long as you can handle it. You're staying above and beyond going over the edge. Sometimes it's like holding onto the back of a jet plane; sometimes it's like the sun coming out. It can be very, very intense, and it's not always easy to stay there.

Patricia and her partner Jim make a strong distinction between an extended orgasmic state, and heightened arousal

113

with a climax at the end of it. Patti and other women (and Jim and other men) have been in a state of extended orgasm for up to six hours. They were good enough to do a demo for me. Jim is unusually intuitive, and can "read" what his partner needs from him: slight changes in rhythm and touch inside her vagina or on her clitoris; laying his arm gently along the center point of her belly as he strokes her clitoris, to help her stay grounded; or stroking her thighs and belly away from the genital area, to spread the sensation of orgasm throughout the body. (Having the woman push outwardly with her pelvic muscles is another way of distributing the sensation.) His intuitive ability is certainly a major factor in being able to hold a woman in a state of extended orgasm.

Watching Jim sit cross-legged next to Patti, using two, three, or four fingers of one hand inside her while the other hand stimulated her clitoris, was very familiar to me. Many lesbians are doing this and create highly intuitive connections with their lovers. If they don't stay in a state of extended orgasm, it may only be because they haven't gotten over the "get-it-over-with" attitude to orgasm that is so common in our culture. During my research on the concept of extended orgasm, Jesse and I had several conversations about it and she made these comments:

As I've thought and read about the possibilities of extended orgasm, I've begun to realize that I tend to bring myself down out of that period after orgasm as quickly as I can. I want to get normal, pull myself together. I don't have this attitude toward sex at all, but I do toward orgasm. I think if I could allow myself to stay in that period outside ordinary reality that occurs at the end of orgasm, when I'm very sensitive emotionally and physi-

cally, when I'm jerking and experiencing energy rushes through my body, the whole orgasm would continue.

Dorrie Lane's experience of ESO is a state she stays in without stimulation.

The extended orgasm I experience is about being in a very high floating state that wavers at the beginning of orgasm. It's the kundalini energy swirling up through my body, starting in my feet, and encompassing me and my partner. It's like a hot flash! It's a completely spontaneous thing. It's a state of vulnerability; you have to have real trust and total ease with your partner. You wouldn't do it on a one night stand. I can stay in that state for twenty minutes or so without any stimulation. I've never done it masturbating.

Any thought pulls me out of it, even just the thought that I am doing it. I see it as a combination of the physical, mental, and emotional: it's a mixing of the three ingredients. I see the mental and the spiritual as being the same: if my mind is able to relax enough to let me be in the moment, then that being in-the-moment becomes a spiritual state. Practicing meditation helps you to learn to allow the mind to come to rest.

It's a gift. It happens when it's appropriate, and it's spontaneous. You can't intend for it to happen: trying to make it happen gets in the way. You just have to be open to the little miracle that it is. I have faith in people's openheartedness. If they are looking for it, they'll find it. There isn't one key — there are lots of them.

Extended orgasm is a continual sensation, almost a plateau of orgasm, whereas multiple orgasms are ongoing individual orgasms; with a break in between each one, and then more stimulation to bring on the next one. However, these definitions are concrete — and the experience of orgasm is not. It is possible that what one person is calling extended orgasm might be what the next person calls multiple orgasm. And who is to judge, since none of us can inhabit someone else's body? What is important is that we don't limit our concept of pleasure by sticking pedantically to a limited definition.

Extended orgasm is frequently associated with tantric sex, which is currently enjoying an explosion in popularity. Tantra is derived from ancient Eastern religions that used certain sexual practices as a way of attaining spiritual enlightenment. But, as you may have realized by now, many women consider all kinds of sexual play to be spiritual, and it need not be labeled an extended orgasm for a woman to feel transported to a spiritual realm. Since no one can or should try to define or label someone else's experience, I have tried to present a variety of experiences with as much flexibility and as little labeling as possible. In the following chapter, I shall explore why a spiritual perspective can be useful with regard to sex and orgasm.

5
CHAPTER

The Spiritual Experience of Orgasm

Sex is about a spirituality that encompasses and honors nature and the feminine. Awakening our sexuality and finding out how sensitive our bodies really are is a life-long journey about finding our deeper selves. — Deborah Sundahl

Apart from the practice of Tantra, spirituality and sexuality have generally been seen as incompatible. All the great religious/cultural systems we know today — Judaism, Christianity, Islam, Hinduism, and Buddhism — require at least separation, and more often, renunciation of carnal love in order for an individual to attain spiritual enlightenment. In centuries past (that is, prior to the relatively modern idea of a separation between church and state), these male-dominated cultures dictated morality, and exerted political control by holding the threat of damnation over those who did not agree with them. This imposed morality often resulted in great suffering. For instance, a sexual relationship involving two adults of opposite gender required the "sanctity" of a "legal" marriage. Without this societal stamp of approval such a relationship was, at best, unrecognized and, at worst, ruthlessly persecuted. Any children from such an "unholy" union were deemed illegitimate, and were ostracized by "respectable" citizens.

In order for these male-dominated societies to remain dominant, everything associated with the feminine had to be kept under control. Women's bodies and all things female — intuition, sensuality, emotions, eroticism — came to symbolize the "diabolical" temptations of the flesh as well as other weaknesses and distractions, in virtually every major culture on earth at one time or another. Sadly, many of these ridiculous notions persist to this day. Reclaiming our bodies and allowing ourselves to experience physical passion can be tremendously freeing.

Sex is very spiritual for me. I feel very connected to my partner and the universe and feel myself to be "celebrating" life, completely participating in the life stream!

I have had sex that felt very spiritual — connections to deep goddess magic, or the stars, or working out past karma.

Sex is spiritual; it is an experience of openness and vulnerability to the mystery. It is nourishing of all my cells in a numinous energy infusion. It is ecstasy of the mystic variety. It is communion with the goddess. It places me in humble gratefulness — in contact with the oneness of existence.

Orgasm is a feeling of being deeply bonded with the universe.

Yes, sex is spiritual! That energy is divine energy. . .

The Feminine

Over the last two centuries, we have become a technologically based culture, and we have lost our connection to the earth, which is traditionally seen as feminine. We have placed great emphasis on the power of the intellect in an attempt to try to rise above our "animal" nature, and we have destroyed many wonderful natural resources in the process. Yet enormous joy lies in simply allowing ourselves to experience being one with the earth. The truth is, we are as much a product of the earth as any other animal, and, as earthquakes and storms and floods and tornadoes inform us, we are dependent on her for our well-being. We must learn to value our "baser," animal, instinctual selves instead of perceiving them as inferior or undesirable.

Some women feel that sex is specifically about connecting with the earth:

I have had times in my life when I feel like making love to the earth — her beauty is overwhelming.

To truly love and enjoy during sex is a spiritual act — it is celebrating our connection with our lovers and ourselves and the whole living earth we are part of.

I experience spiritual orgasms when I meditate before or during sex, and then I feel connected with the earth and the spirit world around me. This is done by simply being and really letting go.

The "feminine" is manifested by intuition, by our feelings and our emotions, by the sense of right and wrong that comes from our bodies, not from our intellect. Good sex cannot happen when the participants are coming from a purely intellectual place: good sex must involve feelings. Passionless sex just isn't worth the effort. When we get in touch with the feminine, we recognize that our bodies are sacred, and we allow ourselves to feel everything — not just what has been deemed appropriate. Although this will not always be easy, you will see a resurgence of joy in your sexuality as a result of re-valuing the feminine — I promise.

Intuition and Feelings

Productivity is paramount in technologically based, male-oriented societies. Being still, apparently doing nothing, is considered a waste of time. But there is a kind of inner knowing, or intuition, that comes from simply being very still and allowing sensations to arise from within. Men and women have equal access to this ability if they choose it, but it is a "feminine" way of being. Consequently it has often been belittled or dismissed. In fact, in order for any of us, female or male, to be whole people, it is necessary to integrate the masculine and the feminine internally and externally. The process of women and men redefining womanhood and manhood creates a balance of power between the two, because, ultimately, femininity and masculinity have nothing to do with external gender. They have to do with energy, with styles of communication, with ways of carrying oneself, with approaches to problem solving, and many other aspects of life more subtle than the genitals we happen to be born with.

To have really good sex, we must be in touch with our intuition, that sense in our gut of what is right and wrong, good and bad. We need to be able to feel sensations in a way that we have been trained *not* to. It was an integral part of my upbringing to deny my feelings, and if something felt wrong, physically or emotionally, it was my job to push on through and pretend everything was all right.

If there is anything I have learned over the last twenty-plus years, it is this: when something feels wrong, especially if it is a consistent feeling, even if it is only small and nagging, then it *must* be brought out in the open and discussed. But in a male-dominated society, if you can't prove something with a rational argument, then you don't get a lot of attention. Just saying, "I don't want this, it doesn't feel good," is rarely considered an adequate reason for not doing it. Yet it is the best and should be the only reason.

We cannot have good sex without being in touch with our bodies, and being in touch with our bodies requires being in touch with our feelings. If we squelch our feelings, we are squelching our passion. And passion is an essential ingredient of sex.

I know I have already said it a number of times, and I will say it again: verbal communication is essential, but I believe real communication actually occurs on a gut, or intuitive, level, without words. This kind of communication creates the wordless rapport that makes for an exceptional sexual experience with a partner. In my experience, if we start with honest verbal communication, we will gradually open ourselves to deeper nonverbal communication.

Self-stimulation — our relationship to our own bodies — is a very important practice, but human beings are naturally gregarious and we need connections with other human beings. Being in touch with our feelings allows a connection with our partners that makes for two-way communication, and promotes the potential for very good sex.

Sex in a relationship is very important to me. It's about communication and really giving each other something.

Many people believe that the goal of spirituality is to free ourselves from the roller coaster of our emotions. It is certainly desirable to be in and come from a place of love rather than a place of fear. But denial of our feelings is not going to bring us to a place of enlightenment. **There is no such thing as a wrong feeling — there is only a wrong way to act.** We can learn to express difficult emotions in ways that don't damage other people. Getting in touch with our empathic and compassionate selves allows us to relinquish our judgmental tendencies. Being a spiritually aware person does *not* mean relinquishing great passion and desire. It is my belief that any spiritual practice should involve being most fully who we are, and being wholeheartedly involved in everything we do. We are here on this earth to be human beings, not to rise above the experience of being human. And to be fully human means to be passionate, sexual, angry, grief-stricken, joyful, loving, wonderful.

I feel passion is always bubbling beneath the surface of my being.

Separation, Oneness, and Passion

If I had to define spirituality, I would say it is the sense of our selves as not "separate." We cannot be separate from something if we feel passionate about it, if we throw ourselves into it with undiluted enthusiasm. We need to be able to do this with sex. Sadly, in our society, unrestrained passion is often seen as inappropriate, childlike behavior. It is considered mature, more adult, to distance ourselves from what we do and what we feel, and never to show signs of being out of control. The process of growing up could be interpreted as a process of defining and maintaining ourselves as separate.

Feeling intensely was the crime of my childhood and of my adolescence, and I was always told to put a lid on it. I've learned that putting a lid on it is what makes me really depressed.

And no wonder! We in the West think we need to be in control all the time. We think the spiritual experience of oneness will involve a merging in which we will lose our sense of identity as an individual. It is true that during an experience of bliss (which may occur during a particularly wonderful sexual encounter) we may temporarily lose our sense of ourselves as individuals. But we will always regain it. Who we are as individuals is unique and significant, and our sense of ourselves as individuals is something we must maintain if we are going to function in the world. Each one of us is a very precious part of the whole, and the whole is not whole without each of us exactly as we are, imperfect but glorious beings in imperfect human forms.

So what do I mean by having a sense of ourselves as not separate? I believe it is when we know that God is not an external concept; it is when we recognize that God is who we really are, that God is in everything. It is an experience of ourselves as an invaluable part of the whole. It is an experience of ourselves as whole, complete, and perfect. It is when we see the barriers between us as false, and we cease to judge what is good or beautiful. It is when we simply accept what is, and what is feels absolutely right, and we are an integral part of it. Sex can bring us to a place where we feel this blissful sense of merging.

When I have a really good orgasm, I lose a sense of my limited self and feel connected to something greater.

Sex can be spiritual in the sense of experiencing a feeling of union with one's partner, that you both are part of something bigger. Sometimes with sex I have that "cosmic bond" feeling so common to acid trips.

The concept of "something greater" can be called by a variety of names. This is a quote from a man:

I whispered, "You can't fool me; you're not making love to me, you're making love to God!" Her answer was a wonderful "Yeeeeeeeeeeeeeeeeeeees."

A sense of oneness can be experienced for no apparent reason other than a sudden awareness of beauty and joy. Or a sudden experience of oneness can bring a deep sense of beauty and joy. Whichever way round, this sense of beauty is often what gives rise to the spontaneous orgasms described in the previous chapter.

I consider myself to be a deeply spiritual person although I don't adhere to any specific religious creed. My spirituality is made manifest by my belief in the existence of a meaning to life. I believe there has to be a higher purpose to life than just getting through it from day to day without getting sick or losing your job or having an accident. I believe the earth is a living, evolving entity made up of the consciousness of all the beings who exist on it, including rocks and trees and animals and water and . . . I believe in a power much higher than any we bestow on the highest government officials, and I believe that higher power exists within myself and within you. Learning to access this power is part of our purpose in being here on earth in a physical form. I believe the majority of the things that affect us are not necessarily tangible or physical, but are different forms of energy such as feelings and psychic connections. And I believe that sex can be a bridge between the physical and the spiritual.

Everyone has his or her own experience of what life is and what life is about, so whether or not you agree with me really isn't relevant. However you explain it to yourself is fine. I hope that you experience sex as one way of attaining very deep and real joy. And for that reason alone it is worth doing. In my opinion, *any* deep experience of joy is spiritual and may also be sexual.

I was born pansexual. It was simple; I loved everything eroti-cally, sensuously, simply, and with all my complex senses. I'm still pansexual but it's not so physically enacted. My pansexual response is in the act of wonder, of delighting in the exact being of any person or thing that I love. When I admire the sparkling mist on my cat's long black fur I am sexual in my wonder.

Anna Marti, an intimacy coach and sex and spirit healer, says:

We've moved from the 'functional sex' of the seventies where the emphasis was on achieving orgasm or erection, to an inquiry into sex that has meaning.

Many women have a hard time with sex for the sake of sex, and they are looking for a higher purpose — a spiritual connection.

Tantra

Here in the West, the study of Tantra has gone from being obscure, esoteric, and scholarly to being the hottest topic around. Tantric sex is seen by some as the institutionalized spiritualization of sex. It is big business here in the United States, with all kinds of people teaching it, some of them wonderful and others who are charlatans. Traditional Tantra comes from ancient Buddhist and Hindu texts, and involves an immensely complex body of spiritual knowledge and practice. In its original form it was a series of rituals and practices which were designed to benefit an individual's health, and ultimately promote union with the Divine. The central idea is to raise the **kundalini**, or dormant life-force energy within us, which is often depicted as a serpent lying coiled at the base of the spine. Raising the kundalini, so that it flows upwards through the body and finally out through the top of the head, can be achieved by conscious focus of the breath and also via the energy flow that is kindled during sexual excitement.

Because, in the West, Tantra is so often reduced to its sexual aspects, it is frequently touted as the quick way to achieve sexual ecstasy. The true path of Tantra, like any spiritual path, involves a deep commitment to examining ourselves and our ways of being in the world; the goal is not to have great sex, it is to achieve enlightenment through sexual activity. It involves high levels of responsibility and integrity. And that's not something you can do in a weekend, no matter how much you pay for it. Be prepared: if you make a commitment to following the path of tantric sexuality, you will make big changes in your life that may require a lot of personal healing work. As you may have realized by now, I believe this kind of work is essential if you are really going to have phenomenal sex, because having phenomenal sex can't be divorced from having a phenomenal life. Incredible sex, tantric or otherwise, only happens when all parties are present and this, in turn, involves being in a place of complete integrity.

I cannot separate sex and my spirituality. My spirituality involves acting at all times with an inner integrity. To connect with and truly respect a lover, and first of all you must feel this within yourself, is to honor the sacred, the goddess, the higher self, whatever we choose to name it.

Be assured that if there are lots of things going wrong in your life, tantric sex is *not* going to make them miraculously better. If the reason you are not having good sex is because you keep choosing lousy partners, or you have no partner at all, or you have no idea how to communicate, learning about tantric sex will only help you insofar as any path of healing will help you to get to the root of what is wrong. Don't get sucked in by promises of a lifetime of sexual ecstasy from one weekend. We all have difficult issues around our sexuality. One weekend workshop may help you begin to delve into some of the very painful places in your life that need healing. But just as you start to get into them, the weekend is over and you are dumped back into your life with gaping wounds and nowhere to go to get help.

On the other hand, such workshops may help you help your partner, but may be little or no use to you.

I have attended two Tantra classes. So far they have only helped me with pleasing my partner.

Tantric sex is one of many paths of healing available to us, and it may or may not be suited to you. It is not a quick fix. *Needing* to experience sex as spiritual (in the sense of its being "more" than merely physical) may be just as limiting as needing for sex *not* to be spiritual. Sex is what it is, spiritual or otherwise. Some people may choose the tantric path because they are afraid of messy animal passions, and they think that sex dressed up in the saffron robes of spirituality will be clean and nice and pure. In reality, what they may be looking for is a way of avoiding the intense feelings that come up for them when they are sexual. Many women have been so damaged by sex that they are afraid of it. Women who feel this way need to confront and attend to those very feelings they are trying to avoid, and embark on the process of healing.

So much abuse, sexual and otherwise, has hurt many women, so that trusting and experiencing sex as a spiritual act may not be possible or appropriate.

Other people are alienated by the image of spiritually oriented sex and the quite common misconception that it is devoid of passion, practiced exclusively by those with holier-than-thou attitudes. While I can really understand this, let me make it clear that sex that is spiritually based is not necessarily divorced from passion: in its most ecstatic manifestations, it has everything to do with passion, as this woman clearly expresses:

My orgasms are much less thrilling without the component of foreplay, tension and, at this point in my life, a spiritual component with my lover. It isn't so much a "pure" thing (I like it nasty and wild, some force and some surrender), it is the inclusion and awareness of the whole person.

There are a number of excellent books on Tantra. Some include complex breathing exercises that take a considerable commitment to master, but others dwell on techniques for channeling energy and developing better communication with your partner. Anyone can benefit from incorporating some aspects of Tantra into their sex life, and you may find it happens very easily.

My partner and I started off working with methods from a book, but then our practice evolved organically from our own sexuality.

Kundalini

The **kundalini** is the constant natural flow of energy coursing through our bodies, and it may be greatly amplified during an orgasm. But blockages can occur at any of the **chakras**, which are the seven principal energy centers within the body. Think of them as staging areas for the kundalini as it travels up and down the spine. The symptoms that we experience as a result of a blockage depend on where that block is localized. The second chakra, based between the navel and the pubic bone, is the center of our emotions and our sexual power. Blocks at the second chakra can inhibit us from letting go into orgasm or prevent us from getting in touch with our feelings. It is very common in our culture to have blocks in the second chakra, and working on their release can have far-reaching effects on both our physical and emotional health.

If we are unable to fully release the energy of orgasm, we may find ourselves suffering from a variety of post-orgasmic physical symptoms, such as headaches, nausea, and the sensation of being hot or cold. Sometimes these symptoms can be remedied by making sure your blood sugar level is high enough, and you are sufficiently hydrated. But if the symptoms are the result of "stuck" energy at a particular chakra, then conscious work on freeing up the blocked area may be necessary.

When its flow is unhindered, the energy acts like a wave that washes through us, clearing out obstacles in its path. Many women experience orgasm as a feeling of opening and a cleansing on many levels. The seventh chakra, located at the top of our heads, is the chakra that connects us to divine energy. An orgasm that comes flooding up through the body and out the crown of our heads often leaves us with an experience of oneness with the universe. Learning to let an orgasm fill up your whole being brings with it a unique sense of rejuvenation.

It's as if sex is what charges my batteries and I can run for a good long while when I've got a good charge, but only so long. Being in a nonsexual place is not good for me, it's like cutting me off from my life energy, from my energy source. It's cutting myself off from the most real, deepest part of me, the real true me.

The third chakra is the center of the will; it is concerned with power and control. An individual may use the willpower of the third chakra to prevent the orgasmic energy from rising up, to protect the heart (the fourth chakra) from the overwhelming emotions that sometimes accompany an orgasm. If sexual energy is prevented from rising to the heart, you may have difficulty connecting sex with love. You may make a conscious choice to remove the block, and use the energy of orgasm to wash the block away.

Directing energy is very simple: just focus your attention on wherever you want it to go, as you feel yourself approaching the crest of the wave of orgasm. You need not do this with a lover; in fact, it may be easier to do it on your own, at least to begin with. You can prolong the experience by stopping yourself at the point just before going over. As you practice you will be able to stay in that state of "suspended" ecstasy for long periods.

I'm aware of the energy rising, and I use techniques to help it rise. I place one hand on my clitoris, and then I touch each of the other six chakra centers, one by one, very slowly, my head last. That way the energy goes out the top of my head when I come. It's very much a spiritual experience.

The Breath

The single most important key to sex that I've yet discovered is conscious rhythmic breathing — the more you breathe the more you feel, and the more you come alive. . . Many of us breathe only enough to survive but not to live fully. Deep breathing is a door to waking up, to healing and to more personal freedom. — Annie Sprinkle

Working with the breath is an important part of tantric exercises and kundalini yoga. Breath is more than just air; it oxygenates our blood, which allows our miraculous brains and bodies to function. Experiment with different kinds of breathing: short, quick breaths or long, deep ones, emptying or filling your lungs completely, long inhale and short exhale, or vice versa, and any combination of these. Try visualizing the breath as energy. Conscious breathing will enhance your sex life in different ways: pull the breath down into your belly if you want to build energy; or imagine the air flowing up and out from your belly if you want to release energy. You may use the breath to concentrate the energy within or release it from any part of your body. But be aware that this kind of physical work may bring up feelings that you have unconsciously kept buried.

I consciously focus on following a connection through my body with the life force energy. It feels different when I touch myself with this intention, even though physically I may be doing exactly the same things as when my thoughts are less "pure"! My orgasms from this are often quite intense. If I do it when I'm not relaxed and in tune, then opening myself up psychically like this can bring up a lot of different and sometimes difficult issues.

Synchronizing rhythmic breathing with body movements can promote deep healing. The following technique was described to me by Jwala, who has done workshops on tantric sex all over the world:

I have women lie on their backs and breathe in through the nose and out of the mouth. I call it connected breathing, breathing in a circle with no holding at either end. This breathing stimulates the lymphatic system, which is where old memories are held. So this breathing can heal old emotional or physical memories. I have women do a pelvic rock in time with their breathing. On the inhale they push their bellies out and lift their backs off the floor, tilting the pelvis downwards. On the exhale they flatten the back, tilting the pelvis upwards, and contracting the PC muscle. The inhale and the exhale are the same length. The inhale pulls in inspiration and healing energy, and the exhale pushes out the painful memories that have come to the surface and need to be released. The PC muscle acts as a sexual pump, and as you undulate with the pelvic rock, the spinal-cerebral fluid is stimulated.

Meditation

Spending ten minutes a day sitting in meditation can calm
you down, relieve stress, teach you to be aware of the movement of energy within your body, and help you to get in
touch with your feelings. Meditation is about quieting the
mind. In this culture we are generally encouraged to keep
our minds "gainfully" occupied and thus distracted from
looking within. Quieting the mind is essential if you want to
tap into your intuition, and if you want to be really present
for anything.

Some people experience oneness when they meditate.
They arrive at a state of "no-thought," where they lose their
sense of separation. As Jana, the Buddhist monk, says, this is
the same place you can get to during orgasm:

*A really good orgasm takes me to a place that it takes me
months of sitting in za-zen to get to.*

Letting go into sexual ecstasy is not so different from
letting go into spiritual ecstasy, after all. They both require
going beyond the gratification of the ego, and this requires
coming from a place of integrity and honesty.

There are many different methods of meditating and there
are marvelous teachers and books on the subject. If you want
to meditate specifically as an aid to your sexual awareness,
you can even masturbate as a meditation: learning to be fully
focused, present, and centered in your experience of sexual
arousal.

Love, Sex, and Sanity

Spirituality is about learning to love. Our lessons in love very often come from the people we are sexual with. Therefore, although it is a concept we have lost sight of in our society, I see relationship as a spiritual practice.

We are rarely encouraged to love unconditionally today, unless it is in the context of religion or patriotism. How we are "supposed" to feel about someone is based on all kinds of external judgments. Parents are supposed to love their children, and children their parents. You are supposed to feel a greater kinship with someone from your own country than you are towards people from other countries. You are not supposed to feel sexual love for someone much younger or much older than yourself. You are supposed to love your spouse to the exclusion of all others. You are certainly not supposed to feel sexual love towards anyone of the same gender. In reality, however, love is rarely so discriminatory.

Love is a way of being in the world.

Learning to love fully involves opening your heart. Opening your heart is not easy if you have learned to keep it closed to prevent experiencing pain and loss. You *will* experience pain and loss when you open your heart, but you will also experience the love, joy, and connections with other beings that make life worth living. Opening your heart may be a long, slow process. You open it a little and then close it a little, open it, close it. A great orgasm can sweep away the blocks that build up in day-to-day living.

When my heart is open, love comes flowing in from whomever or whatever I'm loving, as well as from the earth, the sky, the goddess.

However, I am not saying that if you open your heart, you are going to want to be sexual with everyone, nor that if you are sexual with lots of people, you are going to open your heart to them all. Be compassionate, but be discerning about who you open up to sexually. Just because you are sexual with someone doesn't mean it is wise to open your heart to that person on a long-term basis. The person who was with you when you had that great orgasm (or two or three or four . . .) might have been wonderful last night, but you made the love happen together, and chances are that you can also experience love in other ways and from other sources. When you've just had an incredible orgasm, you may reach a kind of altered state where you are highly receptive or suggestible. In this state you can become disoriented and make unwise decisions.

When I'm with the right person it's easier to slip out of "reality" in that intimate space so that I get the feeling we are both caught up in something bigger than us, which I regard as the life force/source. I don't often orgasm in this situation — lots of intense coming feelings with no real peak — but if I do come it's a definite merging/ boundaryless space of all body/no body rolling and tumbling like a pebble at the edge of the ocean. Post orgasm, I have real difficulty focusing and "see" my lover quite differently.

Whether or not you end up in a long-term relationship with any lover, allow the love to empower you in *yourself* and in your life. I'm not saying you shouldn't stay with one person for the rest of your life. If that's what works for you, then go for it. But this model simply doesn't work for everyone, and if it doesn't work for you, then don't beat yourself up over it. There are plenty of other models that might work for you. They are, or should be, a matter of individual choice.

I suppose one day when I'm ninety I might feel differently, but right now I can't imagine one person fulfilling me sexually.

It would be too exhausting to be sexual with lots of people, not because of the sex, but the aftereffects.

It doesn't work for me to limit myself to having only one sexual-love relationship, any more than it would for me to say I will have only one friend.

It all just seems too dicey and complicated to get into being sexual with someone that I don't have a major commitment to.

In theory, opening your heart is not dependent on being in a relationship, but for many women sex is a way of bonding with their partner. In fact, most women can't separate their sexual experiences from their feelings for their partner. And sex is incredible when it is combined with a psychic and emotional connection.

There's a huge difference in intensity of orgasms, from functional when self stimulated, to incredibly intense within a committed lover relationship.

Sex with another person is about melting, opening, fusing, sharing.

In the long term, sex is undeniably about the way we relate to the rest of the world, but in the short term, sex doesn't have to be about anyone else at all, it can just be about you and your relationship to the forces of life. This is what Linci means when she says that sex is a spiritual experience, and it being so is *not* dependent on her having a deep emotional bond with her partner. We tend to look for someone outside of our selves to make us feel good. Sometimes we get so busy searching for a relationship, when what we really need to do is to look within and learn to love ourselves.

It's easier to immerse myself in bad habits and familiar ways of being in the world than to take the courage to admire myself, to step into the sacred space with myself to see all of who I am.

It is so easy to get caught up in negative relationship patterns because love is so important to us, we may be unable to see beyond our fear of losing it. It is a very real human need, to want to feel loved by others. When we're getting enough love, life is much more likely to seem wonderful. But love from others will never fill the vacuum that exists if we don't love ourselves. We will never have the kinds of relationships we crave until we know how to love ourselves.

The fact that many women don't have satisfactory sex lives is often because of problems they are having in relating to their sexual partners. The root cause may be that a woman has not looked at her own issues and hasn't learned to love herself. This may take many forms: perhaps she is clinging to the lover she has, instead of trusting that there are other people in the world she can be close to; perhaps she wants the relationship to be a certain way instead of letting it evolve; perhaps she is withholding emotions; perhaps she is afraid of asking for what she wants; perhaps she loses a sense of herself when she is in a relationship.

I think I'm actually less likely to have great sex with someone when I'm in a relationship with them where I have all kinds of expectations and needs. Intimacy seems to wreck the sex part.

A relationship, whether sexual or not, is the single most valuable arena for learning about ourselves that we will ever find. Every kind of relationship, whether easy or difficult or somewhere in the middle, reflects something we can look at and learn from, or persistently choose to ignore. If you choose to ignore them, then you will be the poorer, though I fully acknowledge that some lessons are hard to look at. The key to being able to look at these things honestly is self-acceptance. We all have faults, not one of us is perfect, and *we are not meant to be perfect.* Accept yourself as you are and you can begin to work with what you've got.

In the ideal relationship, sex is about love; it is about a heart connection, about merging with your partner, about a oneness with all things. But most relationships cannot maintain such an intense level of intimacy every day. A relationship doesn't have to be all or nothing: it can be somewhere in between. You don't have to move in with your lover just because you have outrageous sex, and you don't have to experience merging with the universe every time you make love. You can love someone and be very close, and only occasionally be sexual with them. Or you can love someone and have great sex, and know that you don't want to see them every day, and don't want to share your household with them.

I had an orgasm once without any direct physical stimulation at all, and it was one of those the-Buddha-came-down-and-put-a-lotus-in-my-heart kind of things. That was with a guy I really trusted sexually and had known for years but wasn't in any kind of committed relationship with. We'd had an on-and-off sexual thing for years. I made myself really vulnerable with him and I had real crush on him, but I didn't feel like I could ever have a partnership thing with him.

Society doesn't accord much status to relationships that don't include a live-in scenario. In reality, the sexual connection, and the love between you and your partner, may benefit from maintaining a certain independence. Moreover, just because you love one person doesn't mean you cannot love another, and opening your heart to someone does not mean giving yourself up to that person. These are some of the hardest lessons for women to learn.

All relationships are games. Games can be wonderful or they can involve manipulation, deceit and worse. — Patricia Hunter

There is a great deal of emphasis placed on finding the "right" person to love and then staying with that person for the rest of your life. Many women equate having a partner with happiness. They are searching for self-completion through the relationship, and they place more importance on maintaining the relationship than they do on their own needs.

I still have the model of monogamous heterosexual marriage stored in my bones, no matter how much I've strayed from the norm. We focus our needs for intimacy on our sexual partners and we don't develop it with others in our lives. Then we become unduly dependent on the person we are sexual with.

It's been difficult for me to love and to learn to preserve my own space.

Coming to terms with the fact that a relationship isn't working may mean allowing ourselves to feel grief. But in the long run, facing our grief will allow us to make changes that need to be made, so that we can let go and open up to something that could be more fulfilling.

Now that my body can get to experience full-blown ejaculatory orgasm I find that what I'm longing for is a deep, loving, spiritual connection. I've gradually discovered that my present husband doesn't enjoy the activities that turn me on, like dancing, swimming, singing, hiking, artwork. So I have turned to other people to share these enthusiasms and I feel lonely with him. My body will still have a full-blown orgasm if stimulated enough, but my heart is not in it.

It is a concept most of us are brought up with, that real love lasts forever, and there is something wrong with us if we can't make it last forever. Real love *is* immutable, but the external manifestations of that love (our relationships) must be allowed to evolve. Trying to control your partner or keep a relationship in stasis may be the quickest way to ensure the demise of spontaneity and desire.

Sometimes I want sex to be just sex, without all the complications.

*Sometimes it seems a lot less complicated to have sex with peo-
ple you don't love. But in the long run, I know I don't want to
jeopardize my relationship with my partner.*

In case you are thinking otherwise, let me assure you I am
a great believer in long-term relationships, although I don't
depend on them remaining sexual. There is a certain depth of
intimacy that you can achieve with long-term partners, even
if you cease to be passionate with them, that is irreplaceable.
Just because you meet new people you love, doesn't mean
you have to stop loving the old ones. And although sex can
be a wonderful way of manifesting love, it is certainly not the
only way.

Some women can have great sex with someone they don't
love or don't know, and other women need that special connection to make sex really worthwhile. Some women long
only for a lifetime partner, while others want lots of lovers.
Whatever you choose, make sure it is a free choice and not a
reaction to your fears. And do not judge others for their
choices. There is no right way of relating to other people and
no path that is more "spiritual" than any other.

*I can have good orgasms with someone I don't know or even
like very much. I don't have to feel taken care of. I just have to
know that I'm not going to be abused.*

*There's something very clean about being with a stranger,
because you have no baggage.*

*I'm always looking for sex that is a psychic, spiritual, emo-
tional union with another person. Strangers don't do it for me.
I seem to have to be in love for the sex to be really good. But I*

can be in love with more than one person at a time, and I often get that feeling pretty early on with someone.

I see my lover as my lifetime partner, and our relationship is part of my spiritual path.

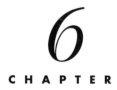

CHAPTER

The Elusive Orgasm

In the last twenty-five years, women have learned more about their bodies, although the feeling still lingers that needing clitoral stimulation for an orgasm is not as good. So the situation has improved, but we still have many of the same issues: women are still suffering from childhood abuse issues, and women are still bringing anger into the bedroom. — Lonnie Barbach

I generally consider orgasm to be one aspect of lovemaking: contentment and intimacy do not pivot upon climax.

I am not interested in trying to have more orgasms or "better" ones. I feel that I've "been there, done that." I'm so happy just to satisfy my natural sexual needs with someone who loves me. If I come, it's great, and if I don't, it's no big deal to me . . . in my first marriage it was made a big deal and I was so miserable!

Variations in Desire

Even easily orgasmic women go through phases when they don't have orgasms. There are bound to be times when we feel like we just don't want to be sexual, and diminished (or absent) desire may last for several hours or several years. Hormonal variations are often the overt cause, although the reasons for hormonal variations are often harder to pinpoint. Sometimes it's part of the monthly menstrual cycle:

My body needs to be receptive to sex, which it often isn't, but the best time is right after my period. My orgasms are best after my period because my body is craving sex. Other times of the month sex can feel like an invasion and I do not enjoy it.

Needless to say, not everyone has the experience of feeling sexual right after their period. Some women are horniest when they are ovulating, and others at the beginning of their period. Terry very specifically says she wants penetration during her period. Many women don't notice any monthly variation in desire.

It is important for us to learn to respect that there are times when our bodies don't want sex no matter how much our minds might think it's a good idea. Due to the pressures of the society we live in, it is often impossible for us to give in to the needs dictated by our monthly cycles. Perhaps the day will come when we arrange our schedules according to our hormones, but for now we are usually forced to make our hormones fit into our schedules, which is often easier said than done.

Sexual desire apart, all sorts of feelings may be simmering under the surface throughout the month and only become obvious when a woman is premenstrual. Hormonal cycles are often belittled with remarks like, "Oh, she's just on her period," but it is important to realize that the feelings that come up for a woman when she is menstrual or premenstrual are feelings that actually exist for her all the time. A woman may feel consistent ambivalence about sex but it may only be when her hormones are really raging that she recognizes it. Whatever feelings come up, they are real, and they are important, and they need to be attended to. And it will probably be easier to express them appropriately if their owner is not trying to ignore them.

Women's bodies change with the onset of menopause, and their patterns of desire may increase or decrease. Even if sexual desire remains the same, some women find that their sexual responses are different.

My interest in sex dropped dramatically upon entering the menopause years.

My orgasms have changed since I became menopausal. There are often several plateaus which seem like they might be a rather mild orgasm but if I continue sexual stimulation the energy continues to build to a powerful orgasm. I can also stop at any of the plateaus and be satisfied. Previously I could move more quickly to a powerful orgasm and my body seemed to demand that I get there. Now my sexual energy is slower.

My personal experience with menopause is that I have just as much or more sexual desire but my orgasms are less explosive and more diffuse than they used to be. Once again, women differ. There may be so many other physical or psychological factors affecting us during this period of our lives that it becomes impossible to pinpoint what is cause and what is effect.

Hysterectomies, Medications, and Aging

Women are likely to notice a difference in their sexual responses following a hysterectomy. It is commonly reported by the medical establishment that if the ovaries are not removed, then a woman's hormonal cycles, and consequently her sexuality, are not affected. But we know that the uterus contracts during sexual excitement; if there is no uterus, then there may not be the same sensations of pleasure. Some women have reported their orgasms occurring in the place where their uterus once lay before it was removed. Other women enjoy sex less after a hysterectomy. Unfortunately, doctors rarely inform women of this possibility. In fact, they often seem to be unaware of this particular side effect of the surgery.

A woman facing a hysterectomy might want to express her concerns to her surgeon.

The existence and location of the G spot is extremely important for surgeons to consider when performing operations. Cutting in the wrong place may deprive certain women of future pleasure. . . this may depend upon the type of surgery performed as well as which nerves and tissues were disturbed. (The G Spot, Ladas, Whipple and Perry, New York: Holt, Rinehart and Winston)

There are many kinds of medical problems that affect sexuality. Endometriosis, interstitial cystitis, and fibroid tumors can all cause pain with sexual arousal or intercourse. Medications can affect sexual desire in various ways. For example, medication to lower blood pressure also lowers desire. All antidepressants except Wellbutrin and Serzone are reported (by the manufacturers as well as by consumers) to affect sexuality, either frequently or occasionally. One doctor I spoke with said that thirteen to twenty-six percent of women taking

Prozac-related antidepressants will suffer from anorgasmia as a result. Patients are seldom informed of this side effect, since doctors are reluctant to discourage them from taking the medication. Some people don't notice anything, but others experience a wide variety of effects, from increase or lessening of desire to different sorts of sexual dysfunction. Lisa describes her experience on Prozac:

The medication affects my timing: when the action is really hot, and I'm having passionate sex and I want to come, I can't, then when the party is over I have an orgasm, but it's really too late. There have been times when I've had to work so hard for an orgasm that it just really wasn't worth it.

It is often assumed that older women have less sexual desire, but this is by no means always true. The women I spoke with who were over sixty had all noticed changes but not always a decrease in desire. Some women find that they feel freer to be themselves and better able to express their passion as they get older.

I think that in spite of the volatile passions of young womanhood, age has brought me the real gift of passion. I love its physical surge, I love that it comes surging out of me when I think the lid is on.

Disappearing Orgasms

Almost all the women I spoke with have had the experience at one time or another of a disappearing orgasm; the energy gets to a peak, from which it normally floods through the body, and instead of doing so, it just isn't there any more. Donna says it's almost as though the orgasm implodes. It doesn't bother her because she has orgasms easily. But for women who don't come as easily, it can be frustrating when they fizzle out, or when they just don't quite seem to get there.

Sometimes I get to a peak but fail to go over the edge into orgasm. Since being at that peak is a wonderful experience in itself, I usually don't mind that I don't go over the edge, and I enjoy retaining the sensations of arousal. It was more frustrating back in the days when I wasn't sure I would be able to come at all. On a mental level I wanted to have something I could be sure was really an orgasm, and I wanted my partner to feel that she had satisfied me. Nowadays I have orgasms more easily, but I don't depend on them for satisfaction.

A number of women said they weren't always certain whether they were coming or not, which suggests that the boundaries between orgasm and being highly charged sexually — almost coming, on the edge of coming — are somewhat blurred. I know that I have had the experience of not being sure whether what just happened was an orgasm or not, and it really doesn't matter, because I no longer need to put a label on it. An orgasm can vary from a full-blown explosion that leaves you feeling totally relaxed, to what Clara calls an almost-asm, which is a kind of a peak but without any real release. Orgasms can have a long buildup and then slowly fade away to nothing without any kind of explosion, or they can come very fast and be gone just as swiftly. There may be very little experience of a peak, simply a sense of excitement followed by a sense of relaxation. There may be a very clear and definite peak, or there may be no experience of a peak. And there are many variations in between.

Recognizing an Orgasm

An orgasm may be so mild that we don't realize that what we are experiencing deserves that label. Sometimes what it takes for us to recognize orgasms is for someone else to tell us that it seems as though we are having them. We can train ourselves to feel something physically, when we have a mental assurance that it exists.

So how *do* you know? Some say that you can tell when you've had an orgasm because there is a sense of ending, a culmination, and you stop desiring more sex. This may be a way of divining the difference between what is an orgasm and what isn't, if you have very mild ones. If you masturbate regularly and have not experienced anything you would label as an orgasm, then ask yourself what it is that makes you decide to stop masturbating. If the answer is, "Why would I go on?" then you are probably having very mild orgasms. Don't worry: with a little time and concentration you will very likely build up to bigger ones.

It is true that some women have one big orgasm and that's it, they don't want to be touched any more. But just as many women claim that they can come all night, which doesn't fit with the idea of an orgasm being the point where desire ceases. Other women (such as myself) need to have multiple orgasms before we feel satisfied: having just one is going over the top, but only just, and it does not involve a cessation of desire.

It is also not uncommon for a woman to feel overwhelmed by the desire to stop being sexual when she has *not* had an orgasm. Laura used to think that orgasms were overrated because she always arrived at a point during lovemaking when she suddenly stopped wanting sex. She thought that cessation of desire was an orgasm, because it certainly was an ending for her.

I'd try and try and try to stay with my sexual desire until he came, for his sake, but then I'd hit a wall and I'd start crying, because I just couldn't go on any more.

Other women say that sometimes the sensation of being penetrated quite suddenly becomes too much for them.

Sometimes with penetration, the excitement can build and then I'll suddenly feel satiated, or that I just can't take any more.

The feeling of "stop now!" is not necessarily connected with orgasm at all, in fact it may not even be a physical reaction. Instead, it may be a feeling of anxiety that surfaces without warning from the unconscious.

Anorgasmic Women

How many women really don't have orgasms? Probably many more than we realize, since it's hard for a woman to admit she doesn't have them. I had questionnaires from ninety-five women, and I personally spoke with thirty more women. Of these one hundred twenty-five, six of them (aged twenty-three, twenty-eight, thirty-six, forty-one, forty-seven, and fifty-nine) were anorgasmic, one (aged sixty-two) wasn't sure, and one didn't have an orgasm till she was forty-one. Several women said they were dissatisfied with their sexual responses: one said she didn't think she was experiencing her full potential of orgasm; another was frustrated because she couldn't have orgasms with her boyfriend, only on her own. It is notable that the majority of women who filled in the questionnaire were in their thirties and forties. I think there are many teenagers who don't have orgasms, and aren't going to talk about it. I only heard from three women under twenty, all of whom were orgasmic. Although there is far more real information available about sex these days than there was twenty or thirty years ago, people have to *want* to find it, and in some ways there is less encouragement to look for it than there was ten years ago (perhaps because of fear of AIDS, perhaps because of the backlash against the sexual revolution of the seventies).

There are probably also a number of older women who are not having orgasms because they are from a generation that didn't experiment much, due to fewer options and less efficient methods of birth control. Uncooperative partners may always be a problem.

My husband didn't appreciate my need for clitoral stimulation during intercourse. I think he felt like vaginal stimulation from him should be sufficient. He said I was too demanding.

On the other hand, some older women are having better sex than they were earlier on in life.

Now that I'm fifty I expect to have orgasms when I'm making love, even multiple orgasms. But I wouldn't have expected to have an orgasm with my lover in my twenties.

This may be biological, it may be a matter of the self confidence that comes with age, or it may be thanks to greater access to birth control. Most likely it is because sex (and life in general) is a learned activity that gets better with practice. Speaking from my own experience, some of us just get less uptight as we get older, as we begin to heal from the negative effects of our repressive childhoods.

As I've said earlier, I never intended my survey to be statistically viable. However, other surveys do claim to be statistically sound. I am a little suspicious of such claims because I think women won't say anything at all if they don't have orgasms. Therefore I believe we're only hearing from the ones who do orgasm.

If a woman is ashamed of being anorgasmic she's not likely to say it to anyone, especially eye to eye. — Lonnie Barbach

For what it's worth, the 1993 NHSLS survey says that only 29 percent of women regularly have an orgasm with a partner. A survey done in 1995 (by Janet Lever, Ph.D) and published in *The Advocate*, indicates that 83 percent of lesbians have orgasms with their partners. The lesbian survey was from a different sector of the population, so the two surveys are not really comparable. But if lesbians are more likely to have orgasms than heterosexual women, it may be because women are more likely to have an intimate understanding of how another woman's body responds. And if the couple has a goal, that goal is more likely to be orgasm for both lovers in a lesbian exchange, whereas it is probably intercourse, with or without the woman's orgasm, in a heterosexual exchange.

Rita is a twenty-three-year-old woman who doesn't have orgasms. When I interviewed Rita, what impressed me most about her was her willpower. She has a brain that doesn't quit. She thinks about and analyzes everything, and that is how she asserts herself in the world, how she makes herself feel safe and in control.

It took me a really long time to acknowledge I had feelings at all, much less sexual feelings. I was just really shut down.

Like so many other people, when she was still very young Rita learned that it was necessary to stay in control of her body and her feelings at all times. And because she is very mentally agile, it wasn't hard for her to learn to control the physical manifestations of sexual desire. It may be harder for her to dismantle her belief system and unlearn that skill, but I have no doubt that she will be able to do it. She is clearly a sexual person; she has been interested in sex since she was ten, she enjoys sex, and she masturbates regularly. Rita is on a path of sexual exploration, and is willing to take the time to learn to go the whole way to orgasm.

I asked her if she thought it was possible that she was having orgasms and just not allowing herself to feel them consciously.

I suppose it's possible, although I think it's very unlikely. I know I'm not feeling a waterfall, or an earthquake, but I do reach these intense peaks. They're not satisfying, though. I feel that if I could just let go and go with this, then it would be satisfying. I never can let go.

Rita also talked about hitting a wall, which she has since learned to back away from.

I've learned to stop before I get to that wall. Physically it's so intense, I just can't handle it. I don't know how to process that level of intensity. I don't know how to understand it. I have to be able to grasp it and intellectualize it, and I can't do that. It feels like I'm on the edge of this cliff, and I can't fall, and I'm going to fall. I get all tense. I can't relax. It's very anticlimactic.

The brick wall phenomenon is reported by quite a few women who have trouble reaching an orgasm. There are various ways of working with it, such as: giving it a voice, examining it, making friends with it, or finding a way around it. Whatever you choose to do, it is advisable to acknowledge its presence and try to discover the reason for its existence, rather than to try and smash your way through it.

Rita, with her strong will and analytical mind, is probably fairly typical of the kind of women who do not easily let go into orgasm. I believe that we may use the power of the conscious mind to prevent our bodies from expression and feeling. We build a wall between what we think is "acceptable" or safe, and what our bodies desire, and from a very young age, we exert conscious control to maintain that wall. This conscious control becomes so habitual, it ceases to be conscious and we then can't reverse it when we decide it's time to have an orgasm, or cry, or express anger, or do any of the other things we have consigned to the other side of the wall. It is only when our guard drops that we find ourselves expressing these aspects of ourselves.

I once had a lover who could only come in her sleep, from an erotic dream. It would happen about once a month. If she woke up, the orgasm would stop, so she'd actively try not to surface into a waking state. Years later, she told me she did finally learn to come while she was awake.

People who have been having orgasms all their lives often imagine that women who don't have them live in a state of constant arousal with no way of getting any release. But our bodies are not stupid. If a woman doesn't have orgasms, then it may be that she has found other ways of getting release, or that she is not getting aroused and doesn't need any release. It may be that she can't handle having orgasms for reasons that are carefully buried in her unconscious.

I can't say that I was often aware of a very specific frustration in my body, not having orgasms. It was in comparison to other people's orgasms that I felt inadequate. I suppose I was shutting off. I did have a sense that there was a door I just couldn't open, and the door was not the actual orgasm, but just the door to that possibility on a physiological level.

Sex used to be this peculiar thing that other people did. And I never missed it because there was nothing to miss. I couldn't imagine sex being satisfying — it just wasn't a word I'd use of sex. There was nothing to satisfy.

Clara joined a self-help group for nonorgasmic women in the seventies. She masturbated regularly as part of her homework. The group made her feel worse in some ways, because in spite of her efforts she still didn't have orgasms, but she found that she was much more in touch with her body than some of the other women in the group:

Looking at her hand, one woman said, "I just wish I could feel this body was mine."

Ambivalence about our bodies, and the sense that we don't have control over our bodies, are very common feelings for women in this society, and are undoubtedly at the root of a great deal of our dissatisfaction with sex. I suggest some ways of overcoming these problems in Chapters Eight and Nine. But it is important to remember that orgasms are not a static experience. For most people there is a continuum from not having them at all to having really huge ones—and no one has really huge ones every time.

If I am mentally stressed, I cannot relax into lovemaking. If my lover is dominant and takes the time to wind me down, then I can have a huge orgasm — all the stress is released and I just explode — but this takes a lot of work!

Learning to Come

An orgasm does not usually arise abruptly out of nowhere. The process of facilitating the buildup of tension that most of us require before we can let go into orgasm often has to be learned. It is a matter of focusing the energy. Engaging your brain in a repetitive activity can often help. Some women find "counting down" is particularly effective, but it doesn't have to involve numbers.

I sometimes repeat a mantra over and over in my mind when I'm about to come. It intensifies the feelings. If I say the mantra out loud it helps even more; it might be as simple as "oh, yes, yes," or my lover's name.

I used to know that I was approaching orgasm whenever I found myself counting.

One thing is definite: although women do masturbate without having orgasms, most women are far more likely to come while masturbating than with a partner. Other women simply cannot achieve orgasm without the special kind of stimulation supplied by a vibrator, and often only a very particular kind will do. Vibrators are not the answer for everyone, however. And using a vibrator may keep a woman from learning to love herself, because with a vibrator she doesn't have to touch herself; she can distance herself on some level, and thus prevent herself from being fully involved in sexual play. The real problem for many women is not so much that they don't have orgasms as that they don't like their own bodies, and they are afraid of losing themselves in sexual desire. They want to maintain a distance from the act of being sexual. Vibrators can allow them to do this. So they may learn to have orgasms, but they haven't addressed the deeper issues.

And just because you learn to come on your own does not mean that you will be able to come with a lover. In fact, this is fairly common, and the reasons are usually either that the lover is not doing the right thing and the woman is afraid to ask for it, or that the woman is inhibited when she's not alone.

I can only come with oral stimulation. My partner is good at it and likes to do it but I find myself somewhat inhibited when he does it. I am thinking too much and not relaxing and enjoying the stimulation.

We need to define the problem correctly: it is not that she doesn't come with her lover, that's just the symptom; the problem is that she is not communicating with her lover or that she is afraid to let go in the presence of another person.

Once again we arrive at the importance of communication. In this case, showing is often easier than telling. Show your lover what you do when you masturbate. Have him or her copy your movements. Place your lover's hand over yours as you touch yourself. And then use words to guide his or her movements. Approach this with the attitude that you are sharing your body with your lover, rather than teaching them something specific.

I try to show my husband without explaining — explaining seems to make him try too hard, which I don't enjoy.

Taking the step to masturbate in front of your lover means that you have probably already let go of some of your self-consciousness. But the fear of exposing your vulnerability while in the throes of an orgasm is not so easily dismissed. It may take a great deal of practice and positive reinforcement before you feel safe enough to allow your body to express passion in front of another person. But it's worth it: letting go of what other people think is the single most important thing you can do to improve the quality of your life in general and your sex life in particular.

Sometimes there is a specific fear of what will happen if you let go. Perhaps the most common is fear of urination:

As good as it feels, I feel like I'm going to urinate painfully and I have to push my lover away to stop the stimulation.

Women sometimes feel a desire to urinate when they are very aroused, or when they are about to ejaculate. When the fear is as clearly delineated as this, why not try working with it? What would happen if you did urinate during sex? Are you afraid of making a mess? Give yourself permission to experiment: you could try stimulating yourself immediately after you have peed, while you are still sitting on the toilet, stopping to pee whenever you wish. Or you could put a plastic sheet down on the bed, so that you don't have to make a mess. Are you afraid of what your lover will think? You could be alone. If you are willing to examine your fears so that you can create a setting where you feel safe, and you can let yourself experiment without any expectations of the outcome, you may find that many of your fears are unfounded.

The Women's Movement has brought us so many benefits, but above all it has given us the right to self-determination. During the seventies, consciousness-raising and self-help groups for women shot up like mushrooms, and out of these came a number specifically for women who didn't have orgasms. At first they were called nonorgasmic, then this was changed to preorgasmic, and nowadays it's anorgasmic. These support groups were marvelously empowering, but sadly, they now seem to have gone out of vogue. I recommend some excellent books in the Resources section. But books are not the answer for everyone. If it is human contact you need, then you might consider starting up your own local support group.

I feel quite alone in my journey to try and find why I cannot be sexually fulfilled. I would love to have help in the form of counseling, workshops, or chatting — anything. I need guidance!

Great Expectations

The importance placed on orgasm can be very distressing for women who don't have them. The underlying assumption that a woman is somehow lacking or defective if she doesn't climax can have a very negative effect. Rita articulates this well:

I feel shame and guilt about not having orgasms. I've never discussed it with any of my friends, other than the women I've slept with. My friends inadvertently reinforce my shame and guilt. They make comments like, "I heard so and so doesn't have orgasms," "Oh, the poor woman!" The whole women's liberation thing — we own our own bodies, we can have as many orgasms as we want — that's a slap in the face for me because it's an assumption that we all do.

Fear of being judged is more problematic for Rita than anything she feels she is missing by not having orgasms.

I'm very open with my friends about everything else in my life. I talk about all kinds of things. But I never talk about what I'm really thinking or feeling when I'm having sex, and I never talk about orgasms. People don't realize there is a wall, and it's really thick.

Whether it is about having an orgasm, having an erection, having intercourse, or anything else, delineating a specific goal often interferes with free sexual play, because it's all too easy to feel like a failure for not living up to the stated goal. Even the goal of having a good time can be problematic. For instance, if one partner gets very emotional, she may feel she's being a wet blanket and that she's ruining it for her lover. What is essential in every encounter is that we experience the sensations for what they are: if they are good, we will hopefully be able to repeat them; if they are bad, we will not repeat them, and if they are somewhere in between, we should be able to improve on them.

There tends to be an unquestioned assumption that erections, intercourse, and orgasms are all necessary in order to have sex, yet it is perfectly possible to have glorious sex without them:

I've found sexual play without orgasm satisfying in other ways. Orgasms are not the end-all and be-all of making love.

One woman told me that she used to place a great deal of importance on having an orgasm during each and every sexual encounter until she fell in love with someone whom she could only meet in public situations where it was impossible for him to go down on her. Since she doesn't have orgasms except through oral stimulation of her clitoris, she didn't come with him. And yet, she said it was deeply satisfying just to be sexual with him.

Women who come easily can sometimes will an orgasm to happen, but the key is knowing that they can do so. If you are afraid of not coming, it is very unlikely you'll be able to will it to happen. As Dr. Joan Spiegel told me:

An orgasm is like a sneeze — it either happens or it doesn't.

So you can choose either to get yourself tied up in knots over trying to make yourself come, or let it be until such time as it happens of its own accord. And if your lover is the one getting stressed out, then address that as an issue of its own:

why does your lover feel like she or he has to "give" you an orgasm?

I know how it feels to get tied up in knots over trying to come: you tense everything up and hold your breath — and then there is no release. There you are, as tight as a bow, and nowhere to go. If you find this happening in your lovemaking, I would recommend stopping everything for a few moments and taking a few deep breaths. Relax all those tensed-up muscles, breathe into your abdomen, and then let all your breath out. Once you start up again, give yourself permission to stop and *breathe* whenever you find yourself getting overly tense. Believe me, deep breathing and relaxation can do wonders for your sex life.

Despite her need to keep it from her friends, Rita says her lack of orgasm is no longer an issue with her lovers:

In my sexual relationships recently I've been fine with it, because it's something that I've negotiated.

Negotiation is a good idea for any couple entering into a sexual relationship, but it is especially appropriate for women who have difficulty coming. Make a deal with your partner: you don't try to make me come, and I won't feel bad because I haven't come. In other words, you agree for your mutual benefit (to prevent either of you feeling like you've failed) that you will focus on other aspects of sexual play that give you enjoyment. Taking the focus off orgasm will mean you have a much better chance of having a good time. And after all, isn't having a good time what a relation-ship is about, rather than having an orgasm? If you are not enjoying yourselves, then something needs to change. But just because you are not having orgasms doesn't necessarily mean anything — unless you feel you are inadequate because you aren't having them. Where does this inadequacy come from? Is it there because your partner feels inadequate? Or because society says you ought to have orgasms? Does it really come from you? Or, like Rita, would you feel fine about not having orgasms if it weren't for everyone else's expectations?

The Need to Please

Wanting to please our partner is certainly one of the main reasons that we feel bad about not coming. Unfortunately, this is fairly realistic: an awful lot of us have our egos tied up in being good lovers, and we foolishly equate being a good lover with giving our partner an orgasm. This can be so damaging. Rita spoke about the negative effect it had in her first relationship, and other women recounted similar experiences:

Various lovers decided that they would be the one who would finally "give" me an orgasm. When they failed, the blow to their ego ended the relationship.

Both women and men suffer from this no-win syndrome. The effect of having a lover who really wants a woman to come shouldn't be underestimated. It may be that if her lover weren't so attached to the idea of her coming, the fear of not having an orgasm would lose its charge, and lo and behold, the orgasm would happen. It may also be that on a subconscious level, a woman may not want to feel vulnerable to someone who experiences her vulnerability as a boost to their ego, as an enhancement of their sense of power in the world.

It isn't always easy to persuade your lovers that you don't want them to try to give you an orgasm. I have had to be very firm about this, and even several weeks into a relationship, I have often had to reassure my lover that not having a massive orgasm has nothing to do with whether I'm physically satisfied.

There is still a fairly prevalent myth that women "should" come during vaginal penetration, and many heterosexual women still believe there is something wrong with them if they don't come during intercourse. Yet most women need direct clitoral stimulation to bring them to orgasm, and only a small percentage of women are built so that the clitoris will be stimulated during intercourse. Either God made a mistake or it was intended to be this way. Dr. Joan Spiegel says:

The way to deal with this is education. I tell them that 75 percent of women don't come during intercourse. I show them where the clitoris is, and they quickly realize that it's not going to be stimulated during intercourse.

Some of the women I spoke with said they had had difficult sexual encounters with women who didn't orgasm. Jana complained that all the attention of the lovemaking focused on the other woman, so that she ended up getting left out. Of course, she may not have asked for what she wanted. However, some women are hard to negotiate with, and may simply not value another person's needs.

Women who are uptight sexually shut me down. I can't deal with another woman's resistance. It destroys my own confidence, and I can't overcome my own fear of failure.

It is very unfortunate that we tend to label someone who doesn't have an easily identifiable orgasmic response as sexually uptight. The two are certainly not synonymous.

Faking Orgasm

In view of this pressure on women to have orgasms, it should not be surprising that so many women fake it.

So many men are threatened, in their own sense of self, if they feel they cannot make you come.

I do it because I don't want to continue lovemaking, but I don't want to hurt my spouse.

I did it when I was young, self-conscious, knew I wouldn't come, and wished they'd stop trying so hard.

Sometimes I fake it to see if I can fool the other person, or to give my lover confidence.

Many, many years ago when I was very young, I thought it was important not to hurt a man's feelings or be open about my desires.

Fake it till you make it: "I can't think my way into right action but I can act my way into right thinking."

I used to fake it under most circumstances with unskilled but very sweet lovers, but under no circumstances any more in this lifetime!

I faked orgasm when I was tired of trying.

I faked orgasm once to end a miserable one-night stand. If we'd been having an ongoing relationship obviously it wouldn't have been okay.

I felt ashamed because I couldn't climax.

The last reason is perhaps the most common, though it is a little harder to admit to. Unlike her male counterpart, a woman can hide her lack of arousal (at least, from an insensitive partner). Although this may appear to mean she's less likely to suffer so intensely from fear of being labeled inadequate, many women do feel deeply inadequate if they are not actually aroused when they think they ought to be. "Frigid" is a word that has been used to denigrate women, when in fact the problem is that they are not getting the kind of stimulation they need. Fear of being called frigid is enough to make many women put on a show.

Women may also "fake it" as an effective ruse to end a bad situation and possibly even for their own self-preservation. People can become quite belligerent when their egos are tied up in making a woman come. Men and women need to stop seeing their partner's orgasms as proof-positive of their own sexual prowess.

Years ago, I would have faked orgasms with men, if I had known what an orgasm was. Because I didn't, I couldn't. However, I did find that if I acted as though I was more into it than I actually felt, they would stop sooner, which was always a relief.

I have never actively faked an orgasm with a woman; however, I admit there were times when I knew my lover assumed I had an orgasm. If she didn't mention it, neither did I. It was rarely a problem for me if I didn't come, and I didn't want it to be a problem for my lover. I think other women may not consciously fake orgasm, but simply fail to discuss it with their partner.

A lot of the men I slept with may have thought I had come. I never faked it, or "lied," but I was probably economical with the truth.

Nowadays, I don't go to bed with people I can't talk with. I try to make it clear from the start that I am not someone who comes easily, and I don't want my partner to get trapped in trying. In the long run, when we pretend to be sexually aroused, we perpetuate dishonesty, which prevents true intimacy and gets no one anywhere.

The real issue is not that women fake orgasm. It is that we should never feel the need to fake anything. We cover up all kinds of feelings, needs, and desires because we are afraid of other people's reactions. The bedroom might be a good place to begin the process of changing this pattern: we are unlikely to be able to be freely ourselves out in the world until we have learned to be honest in our most intimate relationships, with the people we say we trust.

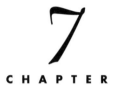

C H A P T E R

Early Sexual Experiences

I had my first orgasm when I was five years old in a strawberry patch, lying on my belly and only barely moving. I felt guilty.

The first time I came it was like a flower opening up, with all these intense, brilliant colors.

When I was twenty-two or twenty-three, I'd read about orgasms but not had them. I figured I'd try masturbation, which I hadn't done previously. The second or third try I suddenly was rather taken over with a "Wow, I'm not stopping — this feels wonderful," and, continuing clitoral stimulation, reached a gasping, shuddering orgasm. "So that's it!" I thought.

I had my first orgasm when I was about twelve, watching a horror movie!

My first ever orgasm with another person was from kissing only.

When I was thirteen I thought about how I could imitate the sensations of sex, and I came up with water pressure. I spent a lot of time having orgasms under the bath faucet as a teen.

I had my first orgasm masturbating, when I was twenty-five. I'd only just discovered that women masturbate.

*T*he question I most enjoyed asking women was when and how they had their first orgasm. The answers nearly always brought smiles, fond memories of such an amazing discovery.

A few women I heard from couldn't remember their very first orgasm, possibly because they had been having them from such a very young age. Or they may have been sexually active for some time without having a clearly orgasmic experience, but they had been experiencing something that was very close to orgasm, or perhaps even a mild orgasm. When they had the experience of actually going over, it wasn't so different from the experience of nearly going over, and they couldn't immediately distinguish between the two. For these women, it was a gradual process of letting the sensation flow, as was the case of a thirty-three year-old who wrote that she experimented with a vibrator and, after several weeks, "realized she was having them." But some women never have orgasms that are powerful enough to be clearly distinguishable from other peaks of sexual pleasure.

Many of us are amazed by our first experience of orgasm. But it can also be alarming the first time, especially if you're not expecting it.

My first orgasm happened when I was thirteen or fourteen, using the shower head. I didn't know what had happened. I didn't know about orgasms and I thought something was wrong.

I wish my mother had told me about orgasms, because the first time I came I was quite alarmed, I didn't know what was happening to my body.

Terry told me that at the age of four she was in the tub making bubbles by churning the water between her legs with her hands, when suddenly she had this wonderful sensation. Many of the questionnaire respondents wrote that their first experience of orgasm was either in the tub or using a flexible shower head. Linda described sitting in the bathtub at the age of seven:

I used to love to take long hot baths, and one day it occurred to me to scoot down, spread my legs, and put myself under the falling water. I just had the most fabulous orgasm and from then on that's what I did every day! It was great, really great.

Lisa was already an adult before she tried it in the tub:

My first orgasm happened when I was twenty-one, in the bathtub with my legs up the wall, letting the water pour onto me. I'd had trouble having orgasms before that, and I was advised to use the bathtub trick by a friend. I feel very grateful to her. It was like finally getting what I was after. I loved it.

Plenty of children grew up without convenient sources of running water beneath which they could position themselves, or else they didn't think about that potential, but there are many other ways of stimulating the right spot.

I was eight the first time I had an orgasm, watching a cowboy show on TV and using my pillow for a horse!

Now we know why so many kids squirm around so much, and why grown-ups are always trying to make them sit still! Victoria and Marya were both seven years old and both climbing poles.

I was climbing a pole on a swingset and suddenly I got this plea-surable and powerful sensation. It was a complete, very strong body orgasm. I wanted that feeling again, and I squirmed about on the pole, then felt very self-conscious. I told someone I liked climbing the pole and they said, "Yeah, we could tell." After that I investigated the place between my legs where I figured the sen-sation had come from, and found my feel-good spot, as I called it. I played with it regularly.

It was very different from any other time I climbed a pole! It felt great. From then on I regularly climbed poles and ropes and doors to masturbate. Then when I was twelve, I saw some boys feeling up another girl in class, so I started touching myself and fantasizing about the boys touching me, and I discovered that was an easier way of coming.

Come to think of it, I remember now what fun it was slid-ing down those thick wooden banisters in big old houses.

Jana was nine years old, thinking about her favorite teacher at school:

I was just lying there in bed thinking about Miss Paterson and all of a sudden I had this wonderful feeling. After that I had an occasional orgasm from touching myself.

Linci was eleven when she discovered a new sensation:

I was always rubbing on things, and one day something hap-pened! I masturbated regularly. I shared a bed with my two sis-ters and it was a great thrill to be in bed with them and not wake them up while I masturbated.

At six years old, Judy was touching herself in bed when she experienced an intensely pleasurable sensation. She tried it again the next night and the same thing happened, so from then on she masturbated every night.

Elizabeth learned to masturbate when she was six while waiting for a teacher to take her to the toilet. Because she was desperate to have a pee, she was crossing her legs tightly, and found that it felt really good. From then on she touched herself regularly, and two years later had her first orgasm from stroking her clitoris.

Donna was reading in bed at the age of eight or nine, with the sheets bunched up between her legs, rubbing on them without even realizing it, when she had what she called "a nice, fun experience." For a while she was fascinated and played around with it a lot, though she says she never masturbated regularly. Another woman wrote that she had an affair with her pillow; she used to stuff it down the bed between her legs, lie on her side, and wiggle it. She was often worried that her parents would find it and want to know why it was there.

Two women said their first orgasms came through being licked by the family dog. Another told me she was around nine when she first came by rubbing herself through satiny undies. And another wrote of coming while being touched by a boy she was playing with, when they were both six years old.

A Child's View of Sex

Many children don't know what sex is, or they have been told that sex involves two people, so it is quite possible for a child to be touching herself without having any idea that she's being sexual.

From early childhood I masturbated regularly, though I had no idea what I was doing, no idea it had anything to do with "sex." I would rub around and around on my clitoral shaft, just above my clitoris (not that I knew what that was either), and it didn't even feel very pleasurable until all of a sudden the feeling "caught" — those were the words I thought of at the time. Those seconds of pleasure were, I realized as an adult, baby orgasms.

They're just experimenting with their bodies, finding out what it's like being alive. If they're not specifically warned not to touch themselves "down there," they're unlikely to have any moral judgements attached to it; even if they are told that it is a taboo, they may think of it in the same way as they think of defecating, or walking around naked: everybody does it, you just mustn't do it in public.

Many girls don't realize that masturbation is about sex until they are a lot older, because the fumbling attempts of teenage boys to "get in their pants" feel very different from the nice feelings they have been giving themselves. Victoria, who later came to enjoy sex with men, says that in her early teens:

I never associated what the boys wanted from me with what I did to myself. I didn't like the feel of their hands on my body, and I hated the way they kissed me.

Although many women had their first orgasms by fortunate accident, Jean's first orgasm, at the age of thirteen, was intentional. She had heard about orgasms, and she wanted one. She read about vibrators and tried the handle of an electric toothbrush on her clitoris, with delightful results. It is very refreshing to hear about women who were consciously sexual as children and felt good about it, like Joy, who grew up in a family where sex was perceived in a positive light. By the time she was eleven or twelve she was very interested in sex:

I assembled all the information that I could about it: a scientific manual on human sexuality that gave mechanics and various actions in a dry, clinical tone that I'd found in a box of books in my grandmother's attic; a hand-written piece of porn that one of my young friends had found in her uncle's military trunk and brought to school to giggle over (very male, heterosexual slant with unrealistic acts and strange terms); a "soft porn" book about "nymphomaniacs" that I'd managed to buy at a local convenience store; and a couple of True Confession-*type magazines. But none of this really seemed to apply to me or my budding erotic fantasies, although it gave me an idea of what kinds of things people did together as well as what some people (mostly heterosexual guys) thought was exciting. Anyway, I've identified myself as a writer since the age of seven, so I did what came naturally and wrote my own "smut" to satisfy my specific adolescent needs. As I recall, it was a shoot-'em-up space opera and spy thriller in which an adventurous heroine is captured by space pirates, tied up, tortured by a whip-wielding, evil and beautiful alien woman and eventually rescued by the sexy young hero with whom she falls in love and, of course, into bed. So it was this very personal piece I was re-reading and fantasizing over, when suddenly my whole body spasmed very pleasurably, a sensation that I only later realized was an orgasm. And I wasn't even touching myself! Pure mental stimulation. The brain really is the main sex organ!*

Growing Up Without Information

Most women who are now over forty had no access to factual information on sex when they were young, and many

responded to the dictates of society by "appropriately" bury-
ing, or at least controlling, their sexual desire. Jana recounts
this conversation with her mother:

*She asked me about being a lesbian, so I was trying to explain
my attraction to women. I said, "You know when you feel
turned on?" She said, "No." I said, "You know when you feel like
you want sex?" She said, "Don't be silly, women don't have sex
drives, only men have sex drives!" I said, "But I have a sex
drive." She said, "Well, that's because you're queer."*

If a poll had been taken of women who had orgasms in
America prior to the 1950s you would probably find the numbers were very low. Historically, women were not expected to
enjoy sex, and it was incidental if they did. Ignorance of sexual matters was normal; too bad that it caused (and still
causes) a great deal of unhappiness.

Sari, who grew up in the 1940s and '50s, never questioned that she would remain a virgin until she got married,
although she was very interested in sex.

*When I grew up, the rules were there: you didn't have to make
the decision not to have sex until you were married, because it
had been made for you by society. I didn't know I had a clitoris
until I was in college! Of course, there were girls who were sexually active, and my parents made sure that I didn't associate
with girls like that. They wouldn't have talked about sex, but
they talked about them being from the wrong side of the tracks.*

It is important to remember that contraception was not
readily available until the 1970s. Most women were under-
standably reluctant to have a lot of sex, because lots of sex
meant lots of babies, as well as social disapproval. Sari had a

hysterectomy in her thirties. Whether because the fear of pregnancy was removed or as a result of the natural process of getting older, Sari became sexually adventurous:

My assertiveness and my desire, within a marriage mind you, were an absolute turn-off for my husband. I finally had grabbed hold of my sexuality and he didn't want it. In those days there were such strong stereotypes about who was to be the aggressor, the assertive one. I was really changing, and what I was becoming was not who he had married.

Embracing Our Passion

Passionate, powerful women still aren't popular. Donna and Victoria both said that they find people are wary of them because of their ease with their sexuality and the intensity of their sexual desire. The label "nymphomaniac" is generally used to describe a woman who scares them so much that they can't maintain an erection in her presence. Dr. Joan Spiegel has this definition:

A nymphomaniac is a woman who wants one more orgasm or a little more stimulation than her partner wants to give her.

In spite of social disapproval, it is far more acceptable for a woman to be freely passionate and to have many partners than it used to be. The sexual revolution of the 1970s was not the glorious opening up to sexual desire that it was purported to be for women, but it was a beginning — at least people started *talking* about sex. Masters and Johnson published their research and then there was *The Hite Report* — the first real statement from women about women's sexuality.

Unfortunately we are now dealing with a counter-swing from the political and religious right. The importance of "family values," meaning that women must get married, stay home, and have kids, saturates the media. As Deborah Sundahl says:

Any time women get close to claiming the force of nature within them, society and the church come down on them.

Negative Messages and Sexual Abuse

Without repressive influences, I believe most of us would naturally be aware of and proud of our sexual desires from a very young age. Sexual excitation during birth, both for the mother and the baby, is not at all unusual.

When we are born we are full of our mother's hormones. Baby boys are born with erections and very young baby girls can have orgasms.

I remember masturbating and having orgasms when I was still in the crib.

Children exhibit very different rates of sexual awareness. In some instances (unfortunately rare) they are encouraged to investigate their own sexuality at their own rate without being influenced one way or another. But the majority of girls are still discouraged from actively exploring their own sexuality, and they may find it impossible to locate well-intentioned sources of information.

I looked and looked for pornography when I was in my early teens because I was already sexually active, and I knew there must be more to sex than what was happening to me. When I was fifteen a girl came to stay the night, and asked me as we whispered in bed, "Have you ever masturbated?" I didn't know what she meant, said "No," and she placed her fingers on my clitoris and showed me how to move my fingers. But then she told everyone at school that I had "initiated" sex with her and she wouldn't talk to me. I was so confused.

It is not only girls who suffer as a result of the misinformation and lack of information with regard to sex and gender. One man wrote that he had been molested by an older woman before he reached school age. Once he started school:

I learned that this type of activity could cause pregnancy, and I was dead scared that I was going to be the one who would get pregnant. That fear lived with me for many years because I didn't understand the full thing.

Sadly, there is no doubt that many children are inappropriately sexualized by the adults around them. Andrea learned to use her hand for masturbation from her grandfather, who molested her.

Women's reactions to being sexualized in this fashion vary tremendously. Laura's first orgasm occurred spontaneously when she was watching a horse race at the age of twenty-four.

I went to the races with a boyfriend. He was off placing a bet and I got down by the rail just in time to watch the horses running toward me on the home stretch. As they ran by I had my first orgasm! No one was touching me, and I wasn't thinking about sex, but the beauty and vitality and competitive spirit of those racing horses just took me to orgasm! It turns me on just to remember that!

From this description and from what she and her partner say about her now that she is forty-six, it's clear that Laura reaches orgasm quickly and easily. Yet she didn't have her first one until she was twenty-four, and her second at the age of thirty-one, when her husband was stimulating her G spot with his hand. She didn't orgasm again until some years later, when she began to make love with women. Now she comes very easily from penetration (without clitoral stimulation). In spite of this fact, she never came during intercourse with men, although she had intercourse many times. Why not? The answer seems to be straightforward: she was severely sexually abused by men as a child, and dislikes penises. She never felt relaxed enough during sex that involved a penis to be able to let go and come, no matter how much physical enjoyment she got from penetration.

Being caught masturbating was the lead-in Laura's father used to begin molesting her. As a result Laura has a strong emotional reaction against masturbation, and did not do it for many years.

It used to be that I couldn't even stand the word masturbation. I've just recently got to where I can say the word and hear others talk about it and not get totally bummed.

Women who feel comfortable touching their own genitals are a lot more likely to have orgasms early in life than women who aren't comfortable touching themselves. Most women have their first orgasm through stimulation of the clitoris with their own fingers. I know that if I had been used to touching myself, and had had years to practice the gradual buildup of sensation that resulted from touching myself, my first orgasm would have been a much smoother and easier experience — and it would have happened much earlier. The fact that I didn't touch myself regularly, and had some emotional unease about doing so, is due to my own history of sexual abuse. But I also remember being smacked for touching myself between my legs, so I learned from a young age that no matter who else might touch me there, I was not to touch myself.

Negative associations around masturbation are even easier to pick up than negative associations around sex in general. After all, sex is necessary in order to have children, but masturbation is never necessary. A number of the questionnaire respondents reported that they were very concerned about being caught touching themselves, and absolutely no one said that they ever thought it was anything but taboo. Sometimes children are severely threatened for touching their genital area.

When I was eleven or twelve I was at a Catholic school and one of the nuns caught me masturbating. She took me to the Mother Superior who told me I would be reported to the authorities if I did it again. I assumed she meant the police. I carried on masturbating but I was really careful not to get caught.

People from religious backgrounds often suffer the most. Even if the disapproval is not overt, we cannot fail to pick up the strong social taboos against masturbation. For some women, this may be enough to prevent them from touching themselves — ever. Other women continue to touch themselves but feel very bad about it.

I believed it was sinful to touch my genitals but I did it anyway, and then prayed to God to forgive me — again and again.

I would love to see our communities provide children with somewhere to go with questions and concerns, because even if they are not being molested, they are bombarded with strange, inexplicable, and often conflicting messages.

When I was growing up, I couldn't relate to being a woman at all, because the images of women I saw on TV didn't seem to be anything to do with me.

I got The Story of O *from my dad's bookshelf when I was eleven and read it from cover to cover. It set the standard for the fantasy life of my teenage years. I got fixated on it. I wish I'd had someone to talk to about it.*

In an ideal world, all children would have easy access to people of integrity who are willing to talk absolutely openly and without bias about sexuality. Such mentors would be people with a nonjudgmental understanding of human nature. They would be people with innate wisdom and compassion, secure in their own sexuality. Above all, they would be people who could be trusted not to act inappropriately.

In a healthy society no one would ever have to deny their sexual feelings, and guidance would be readily available for people of any age.

Why Some of Us Love It and Some of Us Don't

How is it that some of us are able to ignore negative messages about sexuality and others aren't? Some children may experience a stronger hormonal influence than others, but usually it is a great deal more complicated than that.

Having an orgasm is often a matter of luck for a young girl — whether she finds the right kind of pole to climb, or the right kind of water spray to use, and whether she has the kind of body that can orgasm from the stimuli that happen to present themselves. Presumably a child with a prominent clitoris, or a prominently placed clitoris, is more likely to come from climbing a pole than a child with a less prominent clitoris. But being easily orgasmic, or not, is bound to have both biological and psychological components. I believe that not having orgasms often stems from the need to exert emotional or mental control over the physical body. But the factors that influence whether we learn that skill or not, and to what degree, are too complex to allow much generalization.

A girl who has the kind of body that reaches orgasm easily may be more likely to experience sexual pleasure early on, perhaps before she has felt the full brunt of social disapproval. If she has already associated sex with feeling good, she may be able to ignore the negative messages, and carry on being sexual throughout her life. Other children just feel good about themselves, or at least their sexuality, in spite of the negative messages, and are willing to keep experimenting with their bodies until the point of orgasm. A vivid imagination is certainly a bonus.

Unlike a boy, a girl has no unavoidable visuals to grab her attention and there is no necessity for her to touch her sex organs at all. She may choose to ignore what's going on between her legs. So if she gets a thorough training in ignoring her feelings, she can apply that training to any feelings that originate them.

A combination of repressive religious and cultural attitudes with negative personal experiences of abuse may be enough to give any woman a strong bias against letting herself go into orgasm. Clara asks:

Did someone walk in on me masturbating as a child, and pun-ish me? Was it enough that all the images I was ever fed of "sexy" women were nymphomaniacs and whores? Even now that I do have orgasms, I still struggle with the fact that I could have more fun if I could let go more. Whatever holds me back is not conscious.

Let's be thankful for the natural human drive to experi-ence passion, which enables some women, in spite of every-thing, to overcome such negative conditioning.

Although anatomy no doubt plays its part in a woman's sexual responses, there is no such thing as absolute biolog-ical destiny. Biology is affected by experience. I believe it's possible (though not necessarily easy) to learn to control the chemicals (hormones and others) that affect our bodies and our emotions, and this process can certainly occur uncon-sciously. At the very least, it is a two-way process: psychologi-cal and emotional feedback affects our physiological chem-istry, and the chemicals our bodies produce affect us psy-chologically and emotionally. The process of being human is exactly that: a process, not something static that can be delineated by science.

When Sex Is Sex and When It's Not

Part of our healing around sex must include redefining what we mean by it. In Western society, sex generally denotes a very specific and limited act that involves a man and a woman having intercourse. Obviously, I believe sex is much more than that. For me, the word itself describes a vast array of sensations and feelings, and may not involve touching someone at all. People have sex over the phone and on the internet, and for some, this can be perfectly satisfying.

I've often had orgasms without anyone touching me — on line, on the phone.

But just as it is possible to have great sex without actual physical contact, it is also possible to experience genital stimulation without feeling sexual. The experience of being aroused occurs on many different levels. A total turn-on involves the physical, the mental, the emotional, and the spiritual. Plenty of women go through the act of sex without even a physical turn-on. Or they might be aroused but not show the "normal" signs of being physically turned on. Women who suffer from vaginismus, for instance, can get sexually excited and even have full-blown orgasms, but their vaginas never relax and open up. They remain tightly spasmed. Conversely, a woman might be showing the signs of a physiological sexual response and still not be turned on because she is not truly present in her body. She has learned to absent herself from the physical experience, and she is not being touched on an emotional, mental, or spiritual level either. Many women have learned to divorce themselves from physical arousal in this way, even when their genitals are responsive to touch. Their bodies may or may not be responding, but their inner core is experiencing nothing that can be called sexual.

Why would a person go through the motions of having sex when she is not experiencing sexual pleasure? There are many different reasons. Perhaps she has been told it is her wifely duty. Maybe she is a child and believes she doesn't have the right to refuse an adult. Maybe she is being raped, and she physically cannot resist or is afraid of what will happen if she tries. Maybe she wants or expects something in return from the person she is doing it with. Maybe she wants physical affection and cannot get it any other way. Maybe she is looking for love and thinks this might be a way of finding it. She could be drunk or drugged. Maybe she finds the *idea* of having sex exciting even though she doesn't enjoy the physical act. Maybe she wants to get pregnant. Maybe she has no idea what sex actually is and doesn't realize there is something missing, but she wants the kudos of having a partner, or partners, and she knows that offering her body is one way to hook them in. She wants to be wanted. Being good at playing the game of sex is one way to be wanted.

Teenage Sexuality

I think many a teenage girl goes through the motions of having sex without necessarily experiencing pleasure. She is sleeping with her boyfriends, or perhaps any boy, because it makes her feel powerful in a world where she otherwise feels powerless. Every time a boy lusts after her body, she knows she's got him hooked, and it's a conquest for her. What gets her off is not so much the physical sensations she experiences during the sexual act, as the heady knowledge that he wants *her.* Maybe her body is getting turned on and maybe it's not, and it doesn't matter because the glory of the conquest has nothing to do with sex.

How do I know this? It is what I did as a teenager, and I have spoken with a number of other women who say the same thing.

When I was younger, I was gathering a list of how many boys I could screw. It wasn't anything to do with sex — it was a kind of ownership thing.

In my first year at college I went round seducing every man I could. I didn't get turned on at all with them. That wasn't the point.

We seem perfectly willing to accept promiscuous behavior on the part of young men, as though exercising their libido is an essential part of their passage into manhood, yet we often express abhorrence at the promiscuity of teenage girls. If a girl shows signs of flaunting her body, she is severely chastised, and dismissed as a slut or a nymphomaniac.

When I was a teenager, people called me a slut and sneered at me because of the way I dressed.

Because I was promiscuous as a teenager and I fully understand its appeal, I do not have negative judgments about it. It may be a necessary phase for some girls, and most will grow out of it. But I am concerned about teenagers who act out in this way, for several reasons. It may indicate they are not getting the kind of love they need. Clearly, they don't have a high sense of self-worth, and we as a society are not offering them ways to develop it. Nor are they getting the depth and pleasure out of sex that they could be. They presumably have no idea of what an honest, open, loving, and mutually respectful relationship is like. Again, we are not offering them good role models. Many adults go through life without ever being in a healthy partnership.

Lastly, they are exposing themselves to society's disapproval and to sexually transmitted diseases, both of which are at best, unpleasant, and at worst, life-threatening.

The Problem

We have a great deal of work to do to heal ourselves and our society from the results of our negative attitudes, not just about sex but about life in general. We must examine the ways we bring up our children and how we perpetuate damaging lies and disseminate inaccurate information. Let me use some examples from my own childhood.

Although there were few overt sexual references made in the house where I was brought up, there were plenty of covert sexual innuendoes. A number of men related to me sexually in subtle or less subtle ways. But everyone pretended that nothing of this kind was going on. I participated in the denial as much as anyone else because I knew I would be punished if I didn't, and anyway I had absolutely no words for it, so I could not talk about it. But I knew very well what sexual energy was. I rarely felt it from my father and never from my brother, but I was aware of it from several other men, both visitors and family members. And so would anyone else, had they been willing to tune into it. What could they have done to prevent it? My parents *could* have intervened and said:

"No, she can't sit on your lap right now. No, you can't pull her towards you like that. No, she's not going to kiss you good night. No, you can't read her a bedtime story. No, you can't take her up and tuck her into bed."

It would have been a constant struggle and a number of people would have been offended.

My grandfather, who adored me, always wanted me and my sister to sit on his knee and give him kisses (needless to say, this was never required of my brother). When I reached puberty, my father told him we were too old to be treated that way any more, so he stopped it. I was relieved, since I hated my grandfather's prickly mustache, but at the same time, I couldn't work out what was supposed to have changed. Why was it okay for my grandfather to have access to our bodies before we reached puberty and not afterwards?

You could say, as everyone else at the time would have if they had thought about it all (which they didn't), that he was-n't really making sexual demands on me, and that since he "didn't go very far," meaning it wasn't physically invasive, it wasn't sexual. Well, of course it was sexual. Why else would he have been so fixated on my cute little-girl body (and not my brother's cute little-boy body) if he wasn't getting a sexual buzz out of it? But whether he was being sexual or not really misses the point. What was not okay is that he was allowed to make demands on my body at all. And the fact that I experienced them as demands that I had to give in to is what matters, not that in someone else's opinion they didn't go very far. Yes, it is very fortunate for me that things didn't go further. But they went quite far enough for me to learn that when a man wanted access to my body, I had no choice but to give in to him, on a daily basis.

The fact that for years I experienced my grandfather's way of relating to me as invasive was completely overlooked — it was of no consequence at all. It is still very much a normal facet of childrearing in our society that children are not offered choices in what happens to them. They are told what to wear, when and what to eat, and when to go to bed. Children beneath a certain age need this kind of direction; up to a point it is entirely appropriate and necessary. However, they are also frequently told when to speak and when to be silent, what to read and what not to read, what opinions to express and which ones to keep quiet about. These kinds of limits can be dangerous when they impinge on a child's right to say no. What my grandfather did to me — asking for kisses — was not really sexual molestation; he never put his tongue in my mouth. But it was an everyday reminder that he could do what he wanted and I could not prevent him. When I complained to my parents, they told me I was a bad girl. So I learned that I didn't have the right to control what happened to my own body. This legacy manifested in my teenage years when I didn't have the conviction to fend off the teenage boys who marauded my body. We cannot expect children who are brought up without the right to limit what is done to their bodies to suddenly develop a sense of having that right when they reach puberty.

Recovery

Statistics indicate that at least one out of every three girls will be molested by the time they are eighteen (the Massachusetts Caucus of Women Legislators, 1997). Women vary enormously in how much they are affected by, and how much they are able to recover from abusive childhoods. Some girls remain sexually active, but sometimes in unhealthy and compulsive ways. Some shy away from sex altogether. Molestation often goes hand in hand with other forms of abuse, and it may affect us on many levels, so although we might be able to reclaim our sexuality, we may not be able to keep it together in other areas of our lives. The good news for women, or men, who've been molested, is that the process of healing brings with it a renewed level of awareness, a sense of personal power, and the ability to be fully present. We probably all have some healing to do around sex, but someone who did not have a traumatic experience may not have the same incentive to heal.

I was molested consistently between the ages of five and seven, and there were many other incidents of sexual abuse from different sources as I was growing up. I began to experience depression in my early teens soon after becoming sexually active by choice. The act of intercourse was painful, but my perspective of the sexual activity was that it was a weapon; I was a conqueror. My self-esteem quickly began to plummet from the internal conflict of that perspective, and by my early twenties I was severely depressed and suicidal. After a particularly violent episode, and with the encouragement of several people around me, I sought psychiatric treatment. I underwent classic Freudian psychotherapy three times weekly for three years. Though I have always been aware of my abuse incidences, it was not until regression under hypnosis that I actually discovered that the cause of my pain with intercourse was from the initial perpetration. Soon after this discovery, the pain with intercourse dissipated. My life truly began to turn around, however, after the psychiatrist cleverly arranged for several of my appointments to be at the local state mental hospital. The reality of true craziness, towards which I was running headlong, shocked me into cleaning up my act. My suicidal tendencies, overall depression, and my willingness to live as a victim rapidly began to fall away from me. I took back my power as an individual and my self-esteem started to heal and grow.

I know I would not be alive today, not as healed and whole, if it were not for my psychotherapy.

I was molested by a couple of teenage boys when I was eight. That was terribly embarrassing. When I was nine I was molested by an old alcoholic at the stable where I rode. I remember I was more worried about keeping him away from my younger sister than I was about myself.

i was sexually abused by at least twelve people from when i was a very young baby until i was sixteen. how have i healed from it? therapy, connecting with other incest survivors, having sex when i want to, having the kind of sex i want, never having sex when i don't want to, nurturing my self, pagan ritual, connecting with nature, struggling and growing and combating the incest dynamics in my family with my mother, talking about it in appropriate and "inappropriate" times (being very out about it), writing about it, developing and connecting with spirit guides, and above all learning to love myself exactly as i am. i spent about seven years being very afraid of sex, but now being sexually active is important to me. since my body was sexually controlled as a child, i feel a pretty strong need to feel in control of my sexuality now. this includes non-exclusivity (being sexual with whomever i want regardless of who i am already being sexual with), a sensitivity on my lover's part to my incest issues (need for safety, etc.), and an on-and-off need to have really good sex. — kaseja Laurine Wilder

Doris, who is now forty-seven, was repeatedly abused by her brother from the age of six onwards, and then raped by him as a teenager.

The molestation really hurt; it was very painful. As a result I cut myself off from all my feelings until about two years ago. I never went out with anyone. I never had a date, and I didn't know what a date was. I never explored my own body or touched myself. My life was just depression and numbness. I thought that sex, making love, and rape were all the same — they were all rape.

Barbara was molested as a preteen, and grew up in a family where sex and bodies were taboo subjects:

My mother was disgusted by anything to do with bodies and sexuality; her revulsion was as pervasive as the air that I breathed. Somehow I started masturbating and having orgasms when I was about sixteen. This might be on the list of miracles! But there's still this really strong mechanism in place in me to deny sexual feelings. Even now I often catch myself suppressing and denying my turn-on. I often have the experience of making love to my partner and not being aware of being aroused. I'm always surprised to discover that I'm wet!

Part of the healing process for those of us who have been abused is getting in touch with our rage at being treated as though our own needs and feelings were of no importance. This may be very difficult since women are discouraged from showing anger. It may manifest in covert ways, and it often comes out when we are with our sexual partners, sometimes in a passive/aggressive kind of way: an ongoing dissatisfaction with our partners, perhaps, coupled with a refusal to take the lead in changing the dynamic. Or it may simply be a refusal to take responsibility for our own lives — a hard thing to do when we spent our childhoods being told we should not and could not. If we were out of touch with our needs and feelings as children, how can we suddenly get in touch with them as adults? Of course we keep on trying to repress them! Old habits, when developed very young, die very hard.

Many of us go through our lives thoroughly repressed, with only the vaguest sense of discomfort, which we quickly put aside whenever it gets close to the surface. There are so many ways to distract ourselves from that sense of discomfort: television, work, books, videos, drugs, alcohol, sports — the list is endless. If you are willing to put up with a mediocre life, it can be easy and comfortable to stay in denial. Healing requires telling the truth, and that can get you into big trouble since so many of us are invested in maintaining the status quo — which usually means lying.

When I talk about having good sex, I am talking about the kind of sex that requires healing. It requires that you have a sense of absolute autonomy over your body, and if you are going to develop that, you have to be in touch with what your body wants. That means you have to get in touch with the truth of who you are and what your feelings are. Instead of ignoring that sense of discomfort (the one that you occasionally catch out of the corner of your eye before you hurriedly turn away), you must face it head-on. You must also be willing to face all the massive array of "unacceptable" feelings that may come up as a result. This is what I call having integrity, which is about being integrated, being a whole human being. It means you have taken the courageous step of being totally honest with yourself. Being honest with other people can only happen when you are honest with yourself. It may mean massive changes in your life. You will have to stop blaming altogether, though you may go through fits of incredible rage as you acknowledge that you have been treated very badly. You may find you have to leave your job, your family, your friends. Your life may be turned upside down. And if the people around you are not going through the same metamorphosis, will not be pleased with you.

I hear the reader saying, but surely I can have good sex without doing this!? Well, yes, you probably can, within limits. But you cannot reach the full potential of your sexuality if you are not fully present, just as you cannot reach your full potential as a human being if you are not fully present. And being fully present — undistracted — requires a willingness to be completely honest.

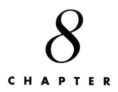

CHAPTER

Relationships

Don't use being unhappy with your body as an excuse to not take care of your body and not cherish it. One of the nicest things you can do for your body is have sex, whether with yourself or with someone else. — NightOwl

Orgasm is a chance to let my body really take over and do what it naturally needs to do, to open up.

reat sex and great orgasms are not synonymous. However, if you are not having orgasms at all, it may very well be because you are not having good sex. I strongly recommend that you do not set out to have orgasms, or to have better orgasms. The key to orgasm is letting go of the stresses and tensions and fears that you may already have around sex. Don't set yourself goals that are too specific or ambitious. If you begin by deciding that you *must* have an orgasm, then you are setting up another source of stress: you are putting your body into a state of tension. Your body needs to be allowed to do what it wants to do with minimal interference from your mind. Try to let go of all "oughts" and "shoulds"; try to quiet the nagging judgmental voices that will effectively prevent you being able to let go into orgasm.

Even now that I do have orgasms, I still struggle with the fact that I could have more fun if I could let go more.

Bodies

I don't like my body a whole lot, and I certainly feel like my body image has affected my sexuality.

As soon as my awareness was brought back to my body, how it looked, how it smelled, the products of it, the essence of my physical body, I felt excruciating shame, utter wrongness. I learned to live as if my body didn't exist.

You need to learn to let your body make the decisions. Because being in touch with our bodies is not something we are encouraged to do, it may take some practice. Take it one step at a time. Just watch how your body responds to different stimuli. Let it do what it wants to do without any censoring. This is generally much easier when you are on your own, when you need not concern yourself with someone else's needs or worry about what someone else is thinking of you. As we saw in Chapter Two, many women orgasm more reliably when masturbating than when making love with a partner. Learn to trust your body. It knows what to do. When you feel its passion stirring, don't try to restrain it. Let it flail and shudder and shake and flutter and spasm and clench as much as it wants. Leave your mind behind.

We are often extremely judgmental about our own bodies. Western culture has imbued us with a deep fear of looking "wrong" from a very young age: too fat, too thin, breasts too small or breasts too big, hair too straight, hair too curly, lips too thin, lips too fat, nose too big, nose too small, body hair, body odors — the list is endless. The most pervasive and damaging of all these is undoubtedly the fear of being fat; America has become a fat-phobic society. Yet our perceptions of how we look are completely subjective: in other cultures fat people are revered and admired.

Work on accepting yourself just the way you are, and accepting the incredible pleasure your body can give you.

People tend to believe that you have to be beautiful in order to get sex, but the truth is that sex (from self-stimulation, or with a partner) can make you beautiful.

When I'm feeling self-hate, I project that onto my physical self and I feel ugly, but when I've been having a lot of sex I can get into feeling I have a very handsome, sexy fat body!

For many women, learning to accept that they look just fine the way they are is a lifelong process. We struggle to believe that if someone doesn't like the way we look, it really doesn't matter. This is a huge subject that is beyond the scope of this book. But being uncomfortably self-conscious about our bodies is probably the single greatest factor in preventing us from being able to enjoy sex. Try to remember that you are just fine the way you are, remind yourself to get angry, and don't hang around with anyone who makes negative remarks about your body. Surround yourself with people who reinforce a positive self-image. And trust what your body tells you!

Because I wasn't a traditionally pretty girl, in fact was very much a physical misfit with my height and size and intellect, I got a lot of signals from society during adolescence that nobody would ever want me sexually and that I was going to miss out on something important and wonderful. I still have a lot of insecurity around this. I'm always worried that nobody's going to find me sexually attractive. Once I'm past that point, I have very few sexual hang-ups or reservations and I've always been happily orgasmic with most of my partners.

Let me make it clear that when I recommend ignoring interference from your mind, it is the *judgmental* mind I'm referring to. For some women, the mind is the most versatile sex organ.

What's happening physically is only about five percent of what brings me to orgasm. The rest is what I'm thinking or feeling or fantasizing.

Let your mind range freely in whatever fantasy world comes up for you. As Nancy Friday's book *The Secret Garden* illustrates, the range of women's fantasies is vast. Don't censor them; they may be a glorious source for your sexual turn-on, and even if they are not essential, they may very well enhance it. The wonderful thing about fantasies is that you never have to do anything about them. You don't have to act them out, or even, for that matter, admit to them. Fantasies don't have to be socially acceptable, politically correct, physically feasible, morally admirable, or legal.

Once you've made friends with your body, examine your life for sources of stress. Many women cannot relax into sex if they are stressed out in other areas of their lives. Find a way of distancing yourself from everyday stresses, and learn to relax.

I've just taken on an ownership role in the company where I work, and I've realized how much the stress of having to generate a large income affects my ability to orgasm, or to be sexual at all!

Take Your Time

If you are going to make significant changes in the quality of your sex life, you need to devote some quality time to having sex. The British condom maker, Durex, recently published a survey that reports that the average time spent on any single sexual interchange in the United States is the highest in the world. It is all of 25.3 minutes. If you live in Britain it is only 20.9 minutes, and in Hong Kong it is only 12.3 minutes. Well, folks, I'm sorry, but that has to change. If you want to improve your sex life I suggest you spend 25.3 minutes talking about it and two hours doing it — slowly. When you have gotten to know each other's and your own bodies, then you may be able to have good satisfying sex in 25.3 minutes, although I guarantee that once you're having good sex, you will want to spend a great deal longer on it. But until then, you need to devote some serious time to having fun. If you are not willing to set aside this kind of time and energy for sex, then I suggest you explore your resistance before you do anything else, because learning to give yourself to it totally is a prerequisite for good sex. So if you're resentful of the time it's taking, you'll never be able to let go into it.

Taking time for sex is a moral and/or religious issue for some women:

I'm sure my upbringing and early experiences had a profound effect on my sexual expression. I was brought up to believe that sex was for procreation only and not for pleasure.

Partners

If you feel that being sexual is a perfectly fine way to pass the time, but just can't imagine having sex that is so good that you would want to do it for hours, then perhaps you need to look at your partner. Are you really attracted to this person? Attraction occurs on many levels: maybe you think your lover is very good-looking, and yet he or she just doesn't turn you on. Good looks and good sex are not always the same thing. Someone you may not initially find physically attractive could have a touch that does it all for you. Don't limit your options. We have all been socialized as to what we "should" find attractive. In some circles this is limited to a macho "hunk," while in others it is a "respectable" professional man. The men who are acceptable or deemed desirable in your social circle may not be right for you. This can be painfully true if you are gay. It may take half a lifetime for a woman to recognize that she is attracted to other women, such is the power of the social norm.

Many women, straight and gay, consistently make bad choices for lovers. If you find yourself repeatedly attracted to people who just aren't good for you, who put you down or abuse you, developing a feminist perspective on women's social roles might promote the changes you need to make. And a good counselor will be able to help you look at these issues. Working on yourself and developing a sense of self-esteem is essential before you are going to be able to make good choices.

Desire and sexual intimacy with someone have often colored my view of that person, to my detriment.

Trust can be a vital factor. Many people need to be in a trusting relationship in order to have really satisfying sex, although others tend to construct barriers against intimacy with people they know well, in which case they may find having sex with strangers a genuine turn-on.

There is something very hot for me about having sex with someone I haven't even been introduced to.

Is your lover really attracted to you? Does he or she really *like* you? It's doubtful that you'll have good sex with someone who puts you down because they don't actually like who you are. You need to know that your partner *wants* to be there with you. It's no good trying to have sex with someone who isn't also working toward making it good, or someone who doesn't want to own up to his or her own issues. If you are in a partnership, you must be able to support one another even when things don't go smoothly.

Withholding Feelings

Even if you are in a great relationship, you may have some unresolved issues with your lover that prevent you from being able to let go. You may love this person dearly and still have some anger or resentment that you're holding onto, perhaps because you don't want to hurt your partner, or because you are discouraged about the prospect of change, or because you are afraid of your partner's reaction. You may have decided in your mind that your feelings are unjustified or irrelevant, but that has absolutely nothing to do with how your body responds.

If my partner and I don't make love for a while, it's usually a sign that stuff is unsaid between us.

When I have had difficulties with having orgasms, it's usually about stresses in my relationship rather than the physical actions.

If your body is holding itself in a state of tension because of an unexpressed feeling, then it cannot let go into orgasm. You must address the issue. **There are no unjustified feelings**; there are many reasons to be angry or untrusting, and there are just as many ways of expressing anger without blame. Let yourself feel what you feel without judging it. The important thing is that you move through your feelings; it may not even be important that you work out where they came from. Letting go of whatever it is you are holding onto so tenaciously may be a very long process. It may involve going to a counselor. It will certainly involve raising your level of conscious awareness and developing the art of real communication with your partner.

I was with this guy for a couple of years and then the sex got to be very unsatisfying. I think what happened was that I closed down to him emotionally. I stopped having orgasms.

A Great Love Doesn't Always Guarantee Great Sex

Notice I have not asked if you love your partner. Unfortunately, loving someone does not ensure good sex with that person. Often the people we love the most are the ones we spend most of our time with, the ones for whom we make many little compromises, because we want to make them happy. Those little compromises may make day-to-day life easier, but they may also be death to sexual turn-ons. You may love someone *and* have good sex with them; or you may love someone *because* you have good sex with them. Neither are guaranteed, and in fact I would advise you to be careful of making a commitment to anyone just because the sex is great. When we are sexual with someone, we open ourselves up to the possibility of experiencing physical ecstasy. This is a very powerful and wonderful state to be in, but it shouldn't be mistaken for an unlimited source of love. Nor is the person who occasions this response necessarily someone you should spend the rest of your life with. Wonderful sex is a wonderful thing, but it is not always a basis for a lasting relationship.

Most people have issues with intimacy and it may have nothing to do with the specific person, but may simply be a reaction to having become very familiar with someone. If your partner begins to feel like family, then sex with him or her may start to feel inappropriate. But this dulling of passion through familiarity may be a cultural phenomenon rather than an inevitable fact.

Maybe you can work on the relationship you are in, with the person you already share your life with, and end up having good sex. Maybe you will need to go outside the relationship for good sex, and if this is the case, you should be able to discuss it with your partner. Maybe you will decide to leave your partner and look for a new sexual partner. This is a choice that many people will criticize you for. We are not supposed to make choices based "merely" on sexual desire. However, the reality for many people is that sex can be the doorway to a path of personal and spiritual growth, and if you need to leave your partner in order to follow that path, then you certainly have my blessing. There is no need to put up with mediocrity in any area of your life.

Communication

If you decide that your partner is not the source of the problem (and it is unlikely she or he is the *only* source of the problem), then the next question to ask is, are you talking to each other about what you need in bed, or are you stuck in a routine with little or no variation, and no discussion? It is possible that if you begin to talk to each other about your desires, you may try doing things differently, and all of a sudden you'll both be having a wonderful time. It can be intensely intimate and erotic to talk explicitly about sex, which is one reason why so many of us experience embarrassment or discomfort when we do. Once you start talking, you may be surprised to find these feelings of aversion do an abrupt turnaround and become feelings of arousal.

You may wish you could tell your partner that you don't like something she or he is doing, but fear of offending them stops you. It is often difficult and always important to be able to say, "I don't like this," and have your partner respect that. The fact that it is so hard to say is a reflection of how much our egos are tied into being good lovers. But no one can do everything right all the time. One person's turn-on can be another person's turn-off. If your partner is truly committed to pleasing you, then he or she will hopefully be able to put aside their feelings of inadequacy and listen to you, just as you will put aside your feelings of inadequacy and listen to your partner. You may want to choose your words carefully so as not to offend, but not offending your partner is not as important as making yourself clear. It is vital for women to learn to state their needs, and state them clearly. **Say what you mean and mean what you say.**

If your partner tells you they don't like something you've been doing, remember, they are not saying they don't like you. "No," in itself, is not a rejection; it does not mean "I don't love you."

Getting Turned On

If you and your lover have not been sexually adventurous, maybe you just don't know how or where to start. I hope this book will give you some inspiration. Talking with friends may be an excellent source of information. There is some good graphic (or not so graphic) erotica and pornography out

there, in the form of books and videos. Beware: most pornography is poorly produced trash that gives an unrealistic
picture of what constitutes real sex between real people. But
there is some higher quality material available and I have
listed some excellent resources at the back of this book. I
would recommend avoiding the real garbage; it may be inexpensive but it will not help you to love yourself. Give your
imagination some interesting material to start with, and then
let it roam.

If you and/or your lover are uptight about sex, and experience shame about being turned on, then you are very
unlikely to have terrific sex until you examine where that
shame comes from, and find some way of exorcizing it. Feeling shame around our natural sexual responses and bodily
functions, and needing to stay in control of our physical
responses, can easily inhibit sexual enjoyment. Good sex
always involves letting go, while the mind has a tendency to
hold on, in an effort to prevent the body from doing something unacceptable. This is another reason to experiment on
your own, so that you don't have to be concerned about
appearances.

*I come easily when I'm on my own, but when I'm with my lover
I can't always come. I need oral stimulation and he's good at it
and likes to do it, but I find myself somewhat inhibited when he
does it. I'm thinking too much.*

Are you afraid your partner will think you look ugly and
sound weird when you are allowing your body to respond
freely? Why not ask? You may be surprised: most people get
very excited when their partner is clearly turned on. Most of

us would prefer someone who is responsive instead of contained. The following are all quotes from men:

*I love it when a woman comes like crazy. They are so very, very
unladylike — it is wonderful.*

*I love watching, listening, smelling women having orgasms —
out of control, into ecstasy — that is very, very pleasurable.*

*My favorite aspect of a woman's orgasm is her loss of control.
For that short time she is not planning or calculating. Many
women I've been with have trouble letting go, but to have a satisfying orgasm, they have to. It's not that I feel I have control
over them, just that they are free for a moment.*

*I made love to one woman who had no inhibitions of any kind.
She was and is the best lover I have ever known.*

Whether or not you have a partner, I would recommend
that you spend some time masturbating. If you don't know
yourself, then you can't tell your partner how to pleasure
you. Play with your genitals. See what feels good. Vibrators
are not a substitute for getting to know your own body with
your own hands, but they are an excellent way to achieve
sensations that you won't get any other way.

Spend time thinking about sex. Note what thoughts trigger
an actual physical reaction. Do certain things make you
squirm inside? Look at what those things are: are they things
that turn you on, things that you find disgusting, or both?
Don't worry if the answer is both: we have been brought up
in a society that thinks sex is disgusting, camouflaged by a
coating of glamour, so your mind may be trying to tell you
that it is not acceptable to feel sexual desire. In fact, the
strength of your response, even if on the surface it appears to

be a negative response, might be a clue that those are the very things that arouse you. Try to be an observer and let your mind and your body do whatever they do. Don't censor, just watch. If you practice this basic form of meditation, you will eventually get to a place where you can make a choice between following the desires of your body or the judgments of your mind.

How do you feel about touching your own body? Do you enjoy making love to yourself? Or do you just want to get it over with? Notice how you masturbate. Do you follow a standard formula? If so, vary it. And take your time! Let yourself think about sex, and let yourself feel all the feelings that come up. Is your mind somewhere else? Are you concentrating on what you're doing? Stay with the feelings that come up when you are touching yourself, acknowledge them, and allow yourself to feel them. This is a practice that I would recommend for anyone who wants to expand their sexual awareness, because you may discover feelings of desire that you would not allow yourself to experience when you are with a partner.

Dealing with Difficult Feelings

We are trained to cover up and ignore feelings of disgust or hostility, yet it is quite normal for feelings of this kind to arise when you get in touch with the power of sexual desire. Feelings of revulsion could be the residue of an abusive past. Or they may reflect the contradictory attitude toward sex displayed and promoted by our culture: while on the one hand we are spoon-fed a sanitized version of sex in order to sell anything and everything, on the other hand we are taught to revile all things earthy or natural. Despite social worship of hard bodies, fashion models, and sports stars, there is a strong undercurrent of abhorrence for the body, especially the female body.

I don't like naked flesh, and I don't like body smells. They turn me off.

Feelings of disgust or hostility could also be an indicator of problems in your relationship with your partner, as I described earlier, or of problems that your partner needs to address. Some people need coaching on topics ranging from adequate hygiene to showing simple consideration for others. However, negative feelings may come from a deeper source. Surrendering to sex can uncover all kinds of feelings you never knew you had. There is a great potential for powerful healing and personal growth here, but it may feel frightening, and fear may express itself as hostility.

The sense of merging with one's partner, or with the oneness of all things, that great sex creates, can also give rise to difficult feelings. As heavenly as this merging may be, it requires the momentary sacrifice of the individual identity, the death of the little ego. And the ego may experience intense terror. Ego, that sense of your self as individual, is an essential component for functioning in the world. Learn to trust that you can experience oneness and still recover your sense of self. I suggest you take it slowly and do what you need to do to reassure your ego, short of giving up your quest for sexual fulfillment.

If you are able to talk to any of your friends about sex, here is a question you might want to ask: do you experience so-called inappropriate feelings when you're having sex? If they are honest, they will very likely say yes.

I went through a period where every time I came, I cried. I have no idea where the feelings came from or even what they were about.

I have sometimes felt the most incredible fury when I'm having sex with my partner, even when I'm really in love with her.

If you repress these feelings, then a free flow of sexual energy is unlikely to occur. If you acknowledge the feelings, without having to understand where they come from, they may simply pass. After examining them, you may find they are not important and you may be able to consciously put them aside. If the feelings are overpowering, you may decide to discuss them with your lover. She or he may be willing to help you work on them, or you may even find that there is a way to play with them in a sexual context. If you don't have a lover, or you are unable to bring your feelings up for discussion, and yet they continue to interfere during sex, then you might want to find a counselor.

There may be a legitimate reason for you to be angry with your partner. Don't dismiss this option until you are satisfied that any lingering emotional undercurrents from a past incident or ongoing dynamics are brought out into the open and fully resolved. You may have persuaded yourself that things are fine just because that is the way you want them.

How to Recognize a Feeling
When It Hits You in the Face

Part of the problem is that we are trained to devalue our feelings, to the point where many of us don't even recognize them. Here are a few very basic pointers for getting back in touch with feelings:

1 **Feelings are not facts or events**. But they are real and they are often loaded with energy. They are *always* an indication of something that needs to be looked at. They often have a much stronger effect on us than facts do, and they color our experience of events. They often arise as a response to an event, although they may sometimes seem inappropriate or unjustified.

2 **Feelings are not rational**. They can rarely be changed by a rational explanation of how irrational they are. Telling yourself or someone else that he or she is being irrational is usually ineffective, and it is an unnecessary and useless put-down.

3 **Feelings need to be expressed**. If they are repressed, they will probably grow and require a lot of energy to keep under control. Try to express them in ways that don't harm the people around you. Instead of snapping at someone who's bothering you, you may want to go outside and run, smash a bottle, or rant to a friend who understands that you are not being rational, and that you just need to vent. Be aware that some feelings need physical as well as verbal expression.

4 **Feelings change**. Often the feeling will dissipate when it is expressed, or it will metamorphose into another feeling

that may appear to be directly opposed: anger to fear, for instance. Allow this to happen; it is normal and it does not devalue the feeling in any way.

5 **Sometimes it is better not to take action when you are in the midst of experiencing an intense feeling**. Strong feelings around a particular person or event may indicate that some action is necessary in order for you to take care of yourself, or someone else, but we are not always able to see clearly when we are seeing red. Allow the intensity of the feeling to recede, then consider appropriate action when you are a little more rational.

Getting Down to Business

Now let's consider the practical aspects of sex. The single most important factor here is taking the time for lots of sexual play, whether you are alone or with a partner. There will be occasions when you just feel overtaken by desire and you leap on top of one another in a passionate frenzy. But if you don't take it slowly some of the time, then you are missing out on something wonderful.

Firstly, make the space and time to talk with your partner about sex. Take turns: first one of you speaks and then the other. Listening is as vital a communication skill as talking. Tell your partner what you want him or her to do to you, how you've imagined it will feel when she or he does a particular thing, and how much it turns you on thinking about it. If thinking about it scares you, it is okay to say that too. Say this while you are looking into your partner's eyes, but if you

need to be in a darkened room with the lights out, that's fine
too. Whatever you need to do, do it, as long as it makes it
possible for you to begin to verbalize your desires.

*Allowing your partner to be with you when you feel nervous
may make you feel more connected to this person. The two of
you will have overcome your fears together.* — Alex Robboy

Ultimately, you want to be able to communicate using
facial expression, nonverbal sounds, your eyes, and your
body language to convey your conscious intent. If you can
only use words right now, then start there; but do affirm to
yourself and to your partner that your intent is to be freely,
openly, and lovingly sexual. Repeat this affirmation often and
clearly. Hold onto your conscious intent, and go back to it
whenever you feel overwhelmed.

There will be times when you don't want to talk, and in
fact too much chatter may block pure body sensation and
empathic feelings.

And remember, neither of you are making any guarantees.
You are making suggestions with regard to what you think
you want. That does not mean that if you actually try those
things you will have a wonderful time. With trying may come
the discovery that you don't enjoy or want to do them. If
both of you consent, there is no harm in trying anything
once. If it doesn't feel good, you never need to do it again.

It is to be hoped that as you share your innermost desires
with your partner, he or she will get excited about the idea of
exploring them with you. If your partner is less than enthusiastic, make sure it is not because he or she feels inadequate
or frightened. A little reassurance never goes amiss. Perhaps

you need a lot more discussion before you can agree on an approach to sex that you are both comfortable with. And don't forget to give your partner a turn.

If you are in agreement, then go for it. But go slowly, and keep giving feedback! Feedback can be verbal or physical. It is often easier to explain where you want to be touched by taking your partner's hand and placing it there than struggling with a verbal explanation. Ideally your partner will be watching you carefully, trying to read your nonverbal signals before you need to make them verbal. But it can be very tricky to read another person's body language correctly, so never rely on your partner's ability to read yours. And remember, it is fine to ask your partner to stop at any time; don't wait until you hate what is happening before speaking up. There may be times when you just need for your lover to pause for a moment or two and stop the stimulation, perhaps to let the energy gather itself.

At the moment of orgasm I always want my partner to hold absolutely still inside me.

Don't expect your partner to know what you want unless you tell them.

Take a Risk, But Don't Take It Seriously

Resign yourself: you *are* going to have to take initiative. You don't need to be brazen about it; if shy is what you feel, then it's fine to let that show. Don't hold yourself tightly — let your feelings be clear to your partner, especially if you are turned on. Allow yourself to be responsive.

It's hard for me to come when my partner is not clearly turned on and desiring me.

Are you nervous about taking the initiative? Then ask your partner, "Is this okay?" But don't let your fear of making a mistake stop you. No doubt you will occasionally make mistakes. We all do, in all areas of life. The important thing is to learn and move on. Don't let yourself be paralyzed.

What if your partner gets so nervous while trying something new that he can't maintain an erection? Well, as any lesbian will tell you, that shouldn't matter in the least because it is generally easier to pleasure a woman manually or orally. In any case, why should intercourse be the sole focus of your play?

What if your body starts shaking or you find yourself sweating with a combination of nervousness and desire? If it's really too frightening, have your partner hold you and stroke you gently. Go ahead and cry if it helps.

Learn to laugh at yourself: gentle laughter can be enormously healing. You will never do everything perfectly. There will always be times when you accidentally pull your partner's hair or do something clumsy and embarrassing. Being graceful is neither realistic nor important — this is sex, not ballet.

Sex is often really funny. Not put-down, humiliating funny, but the "Hey, we're all human aren't we?" kind of funny where people and body parts do surprising or unexpected things at odd moments. Being able to laugh together at those moments peels off a layer of self-consciousness and awkwardness, traits that inhibit orgasm.

Once you have learned to go more slowly, try to vary your pace. Teasing is often a great deal of fun. You might spend days developing sexual tension, knowing that you can choose to go "all the way" whenever you want. Anticipation can be half the pleasure. Expand your definition of sex to include more of what is generally called foreplay. Many women can come or get very close to coming from having other parts of their bodies stimulated, besides their genitals.

Almost any part of my body can be erotic, but especially my breasts, neck, back, buttocks, and mouth.

There is no need to limit sex to the bedroom, but whatever place you choose to be sexual, be aware of your partner's issues. Many people need to feel sure they are not going to be interrupted.

Learn to flirt. You can flirt without looking at someone or you can flirt with nothing but eye contact. You might flirt outrageously in outrageous places. Make sexual innuendoes to your lover over the phone. Send flowers and love notes. If you find these things completely laughable, then perhaps your desire for your partner is jaded. How does it feel to think of doing these things with someone else?

Play games. Dress up. Adopt a new persona or create scenarios to act out with your partner: maybe one of you wants to be the seducer and the other a reluctant (or not so reluctant) innocent. There are infinite possibilities here: the meter reader who arrives while the seductive lady of the house is in the bath; the gardener who is horrified when his employer catches him masturbating in the gazebo; the alien from outer space who adopts a human form but knows nothing about sex and must be taught. At first you may feel ridiculous, but you may be surprised at how wet you get once you overcome your inhibitions and get into the game.

Be real about your feelings. Be willing to laugh. Take risks. You won't die.

All of this may or may not lead directly to orgasms, but as I said at the beginning of this chapter, such specific expectations tend to set you up for failure in the first place. Much of the art of creating hot sex is about *not* focusing on orgasm. It may even involve deliberately forestalling climax.

Sometimes I don't even try to have an orgasm, and it's nice not to have it as a goal but rather just to experience sensations.

I have devoted much of this chapter to the importance of letting go in order to have good sex; letting go of preconceptions, of inhibitions, of needing things to be a certain way, of having goals, of emotional stresses and tensions. The actual physical experience of orgasm also requires a letting go, but in its earlier phases it usually requires a physical buildup of muscular tension. This physical tension is often necessary and should be facilitated, *not* avoided.

The explosion of orgasm comes when the tension in my legs is released and my clitoris pulses rapidly.

Our sexual responses are innate and natural, but sex is not an individual thing, it is interactive. It occurs in a social context, in a cultural matrix, which predetermines some of our sexual dynamics. Learning to recognize those dynamics can help us to make positive choices.

9
CHAPTER

The Bigger Picture

As far as I know, the United States is one of the best places in the world to be an actively sexual woman. As a lesbian, if I was living in any one of a number of other countries, I know that my life would have taken a different path. I doubt I would have written this book, for instance. I chose to live here because I knew I would be freer here than anywhere else. However, American culture is still a long way from being a place where children, female or male, grow up enabled to make real choices, instead of unquestioningly following social dictates.

Upon initial observation, it may seem odd that Western women are typically so restrained in their sexual responses: after all, thanks to Freud, there is definitely an expectation that a sexually healthy woman should come during intercourse, preferably without assistance from more direct clitoral stimulation. But ours is a culture where female sexuality has been and continues to be degraded rather than celebrated. Women are taught to hold themselves back from letting go into passion. They feel obligated to remain in control.

In such a situation, they are more likely to experience orgasms that arise out of tension than out of relaxation, if they experience orgasm at all. That tension, the need to hold back, can cripple our sexuality. Our orgasmic experience might be quite different if we learned to relax during sexual play. Let's look at some of the broader factors that may contribute to this tension.

Caretakers versus Providers

Since the beginning of Western culture, women have been seen as the caretakers and men as the providers. Being a caretaker meant putting the needs of others before her own. Being a provider entitled a man to her care. Despite changing gender roles, these expectations and assumptions continue to this day. If a woman's husband indicates that he needs sex, a woman may well feel that she is failing in her role as caretaker if she denies it to him.

Having an orgasm without penetration, or being penetrated without having an orgasm, or both together, may involve a surrender, a vulnerability that a woman does not want to experience. Other forms of sexual play are not seen as requiring the same kind of surrender.

Penetration is the exquisite "giving in" to someone, letting them in. Oral sex is the ultimate luxury.

One difference between penetration and having an orgasm is that the former can be forced and the latter cannot. This may be why some women's bodies are reluctant to orgasm: it is the one place where they are able to say, "This is *my* body, and I'm not giving it up!"

A woman who doesn't really believe she has the right to refuse sex is going to consciously or unconsciously feel resentment towards her lovers, and she is not likely to want to surrender to them in the one area of her life where she knows she can't be forced, where she is still in control: letting go into orgasm. If she has been brought up to believe that she *has* to give in to the wishes of her mate, and that sex is something that is primarily, if not wholly, for a man's pleasure, then why would she want to surrender in the one situation where she doesn't have to? Especially if she is having intercourse with a man who would experience her orgasm as empowering to him? Wouldn't she perceive such empowerment to be at her cost? Aren't many women already resentful of the power that men have in the world? If her resentment occurs on an unconscious level, then blocking an orgasm isn't likely to be a conscious decision. It may not be in a heterosexual woman's best interest to bring her resentment of men into her consciousness. What is she going to do about it? Become a lesbian? No doubt many women do become lesbians for this reason, and as a result may have been able to let go of their resentment towards men, because they are no longer dependent on them. (But I am *not* suggesting that all lesbians have negative feelings towards men, or that this is the only reason a woman would be a lesbian!)

I think one can see how a woman might, on an unconscious level, find *not* having an orgasm distinctly preferable to having one, even if it means sacrificing her own pleasure.

She might feel she is achieving more by thwarting his enjoyment, than she is losing by thwarting her own. She might
not see it as sacrificing her pleasure in any case, if she did
not perceive intercourse as being for her pleasure. Nor would
she be likely to value her own pleasure. And, growing up in a
society that devalues women, she might not even believe
that it is possible for her to experience pleasure from sex.
But human beings operate on many different levels of awareness, and on another level, the same woman may feel inadequate that she can't give herself to her partner in the way
that she has been told she should. She might pretend to be
aroused, and fake orgasm, in order to protect herself from
being called frigid.

Does this sound far-fetched? Or does it ring true? I believe
that the feelings that drive us may go unrecognized for a lifetime because they lie so deeply in our unconscious that they
can easily be ignored. Bringing such feelings into conscious
awareness is always uncomfortable and sometimes frightening, and may require the direction and support of a professional counselor.

Claiming Our Passion

There is no inherent reason why intercourse should be, or
should be seen as, an act of submission. Many women are
able to claim their sexual passion in spite of their cultural
conditioning. They assert their sexual passion, knowing they
are doing it for themselves and not for anyone else. And they
look for kindred spirits in the people they choose to be

sexual with, opting to work together to develop honest, open partnerships.

Even when a woman does experience sex as an act of submission, she may feel empowered by it: paradoxically, total surrender, letting down all defenses and allowing physical pleasure and passion to take over, can be deeply liberating. Such a woman may consent to being submissive in that context; she may very well be someone with power and responsibility in her everyday life, and wants to experience the opposite in bed. She recognizes the universal truth that vulnerability always requires strength. She remains securely connected with her own inner power, and stays connected to that source of personal power even when she appears to be acting submissively.

However, this is not true for all of us. I believe that the only way to change anything in our lives is first and foremost to be willing to acknowledge the way we feel. In order to honor our feelings and begin the process of self-empowerment, we must to learn to say no. There can be no "yes" without "no": no one can fully consent to anything until she or he feels freely able to say no.

There is nothing worse than sharing sex with someone because we feel we should, or for someone else's sake, or because it's better than not having any at all. I've been there in the past and do not want to do so again.

The Power of No

In this culture, saying "no" is equated with saying, "I don't love you." But in reality, the two are not related. Saying "no" is about establishing our autonomy in the world. It has absolutely no relevance to how much we love, or don't love, the person we are saying it to. Learning to hear the word "no" simply for what it is — "No, I don't want that right now" — without experiencing it as a personal rejection, would greatly improve our ability to communicate with each other. Similarly, learning that it is okay to say it, and that saying it won't end the relationship, would facilitate the process of reclaiming and equalizing power for *both* partners.

It may be appalling to realize how rarely we feel we have the right or the ability to say no in our daily lives; how often we give in to subtle unspoken pressures. Here is one perspective from an incest survivor:

The pressure (to have sex) from my father was violent and life-threatening. The pressure from my husband was the legal and societal definition of the marriage contract, and at that time, I felt that I desperately needed the protection of marriage as a buffer from sexual aggression. (from *Pressure to Heal*, by Carolyn Gage, published in *Lesbian Ethics* in 1992, Albuquerque, NM)

And another point of view from a prostitute:

When it was my profession, I always made sure that I felt okay about what I gave, in return for what I was paid. I bargained for what I felt was fair. I've made many more compromises in my social sex life than I ever did as a professional.

It is not easy to set clear boundaries, but until we establish, in our own psyches, that we do have the right to say no any time we feel like it, there will always be a little voice saying, "I wish I could choose not to do this." Many of us resist owning up to the existence of this voice, because if we give it any credence, we might find it very hard to give in to someone making demands on our bodies, and *then* we would be failing as caretakers, and *then* we would find ourselves alone.

As a young woman, I found that for the first six months of a relationship I was very sexual. Then I would start to withdraw. This was a pattern I could not reverse until I realized that what I needed to do at that point was to establish that I could say no to my lover. I had to stop making excuses, and simply say, no, I don't want to make love now or tomorrow, and maybe never. At first my no's were tinged with resentment because I was still carrying a great deal of resentment from my childhood, and because I expected to be punished for saying no. I sometimes felt like I wanted to have sex, but as soon as we began to make love my desire would become resistance. Sometimes I felt very angry. Sometimes I felt afraid. But when I finally felt that my no's were accepted, I began to be open to being sexual again and I found myself able to stay present in the relationship.

Asserting ourselves is not something that happens in a vacuum. In the short run, saying no, and allowing old irrational feelings to surface, may put a strain on a relationship. Both partners will need to exercise great patience, and tap into communication skills they perhaps never even knew they had. If couples counseling is an option, I urge you to consider it. In the long run, if each partner learns to say no and learns to accept the other saying it, the relationship can only grow stronger and healthier. Ultimately, wonderful sex is about merging, and it cannot happen until both partners consciously choose to be present, in the fullness of their power. And that cannot happen if either partner is afraid of saying no.

Perhaps we don't feel like saying no to sex altogether, but only to certain activities. Negotiate with your partner. Try to come from a place of compassion for your partner's needs, without giving in to them if they are at odds with yours. You may have to make compromises, but make sure they are conscious, and know that you have freely agreed to them. Too many compromises grudgingly made will cause resentment. Make sure you end up feeling empowered by your decisions (it is *never* empowering when you do something just to avoid upsetting your partner). When you're being sexual, stop when you want to stop, which may be long before your partner wants you to. Always do it with kindness. If you cannot get beyond your dislike, or you feel that any negotiation is more of a sacrifice than a compromise, then you need to respect that, and so does your partner. Stop trying to push through your resistance, because you will only make it stronger. (In fact, once you stop trying to push through it, you may find that it goes of its own accord.) Remember, you are not alone, and you are not crazy. You cannot continue to do things you really don't enjoy without destroying parts of yourself, and you are responding to this dilemma in a sane and normal way.

Remember, too, that your partner is not your enemy, although he or she may sometimes feel like it. Even if you finally separate because you cannot fulfil each other's needs, it doesn't mean you don't love each other. A relationship shouldn't be a war zone. It is a partnership in which you work *together* to arrive at a place where you can both be fully present and honest, and both give each other what you can without being drained, whether your relationship is sexual or not.

You may decide that you don't want to have sex at all. Channeling your creative energy into some other area of life is a perfectly valid choice, and you may still be able to maintain a loving partnership. Being sexual is only one way of giving and receiving love.

The Power of Yes

There is another side to this coin, and that is: there can be no "no" without "yes." Some women grow up surrounded by sexual innuendoes and wandering hands that they cannot escape. Other women grow up deprived of any sexual identity at all. This is often painfully the case for women who are overweight, or otherwise considered not conventionally attractive. Verbal ridicule, physical and/or emotional abuse, and social restrictions are typical consequences for them as girls and young women. Such conditioning goes very deep and can be very difficult to overcome.

Our society is nominally supportive of a woman saying no to sex (as long as it is not to her husband), but women who want more sex, or different kinds of sex other than their partners offer them, may find themselves out on a limb. Women who are not in a steady relationship, or want to have sex outside a relationship, may have absolutely nowhere to turn for sexual satisfaction. If we feel like our options are limited, then we may end up saying yes to a situation because we think it's the best we are going to get. We may end up staying with a partner, although we are not getting the sex we want, or the respect we need, because we are afraid of getting no sex at all. We may find ourselves toning down our passion so as to avoid alienating our partner. We may be accused of harassing our partner. We may be accused of nymphomania or sex addiction. Masturbation is a useful stopgap, but it doesn't fill the very real need for human contact.

Should you find yourself in this kind of position, I would encourage you to consider that you *do* have options. The likelihood that there are people somewhere who will appreciate what you have to offer is very high; the question you need to address is how to find them.

Whether you find yourself needing to establish a yes or a no, compassion and honesty are essential for both you and your partner. Although anger is a natural reaction to long periods of failing to have your needs validated (and feelings of anger should not be denied), in the long run, blaming your partner isn't going to help — she or he is also a product of cultural conditioning, after all. Talking with friends, or other people who have been through similar difficulties, getting objective feedback and support, can make a world of difference.

Ultimately, the solution lies in the demystification of sex. If sexual desire were an acceptable topic for discussion, I believe we would recognize and deal with our issues around sex more easily. Fewer of us would get into relationships where, a year or so down the road, we find we're completely incompatible. The parameters for entering into a relationship would reflect real needs rather than surface attraction.

Often the problem seems to be that one partner needs to feel that she or he can control the other partner's expression of passion. Strong sexual energy can feel alarming, especially to people who were molested as children. This kind of dynamic can be addressed within the context of sexual play.

It used to be that I would feel like an abuser if I really let my passion show. There didn't seem to be any way around it. My lover just didn't like the way I moved when I got to a certain level of arousal. Finally we negotiated that we would take turns being the one in charge, being the one to give or the one to take. This works really well because I know there is no possibility of her being overwhelmed by my sexual energy when she is in charge because she directs the action. She can tell me to lie still if she wants.

One woman told me that she solves this dilemma by tying her lover up. Then there is no question who is in charge, and her partner never has to worry about restraining his desire because it is restrained for him. What a simple way to deal with a problem that might otherwise destroy a relationship.

Asserting Ourselves

It is so easy to let things slide, to maintain our lives and relationships the way they always have been, rather than taking the steps to change things for the better. Failing to say no or to take the initiative when you've never done either before may not seem like a problem. But it is a problem if it means that you are enduring mediocrity in your life. And it is most definitely a problem if you are blaming someone else for that mediocrity. What happens is a common dynamic between couples: a woman isn't happy with the relationship but it doesn't really occur to her that she can change it, or the effort of changing it seems too overwhelming, so she does nothing, but still feels resentful. She may end up blaming her partner for her sense of powerlessness because that is less risky than taking her power herself. If she has ten children and an abusive husband who controls all the money, she must be very careful not to incite him to violence. But in this country, many women are in a position to take their power, and what prevents them is not so much real fear as it is the habit of abdicating responsibility.

Of course, this relationship dynamic may be reversed, with the male partner being the one to abdicate responsibility.

I believe that if you want to be sexually fulfilled, at some point in your lifetime you need to take charge and make sex into a form of play where you make the rules and call the shots, doing only what you want to do and what gives you pleasure. If at the end of the day you have only stroked your lover's back, and you feel fulfilled by that, you can feel confident that you owe nothing more. Sex should never, even inadvertently, be a violation. No matter how many times you say "I don't want to do anything that you don't want to," if you never say, "Okay, this is what I want," then the relationship can never grow. Whether it is sleeping alone, having separate beds, doing nothing explicitly sexual, masturbating across the room while your partner watches, or vice versa, doing cunnilingus and nothing else, engaging in sex only in a spiritual context — whatever it is, no matter how seemingly radical, you must decide what it is you really want and negotiate with your partner from there.

Once you have learned to take charge, you can make the conscious choice *not* to be in charge if that's what you want. And remember, changing your mind is always an option.

Do sex the way you want to do it, and know that you are doing it because you have chosen it. The best partners are the ones who are doing it for themselves, from a place of compassion and openheartedness. When I asked Jesse how she would describe to someone how to give her oral sex, she said:

I wouldn't tell somebody how to give me oral sex. That would be like telling someone how to talk to me, what to say to me. I want to hear what they have to say.

This is a very astute observation and explains why sex manuals often come up short. What is needed is not so much information on the practical aspects of sex, but more information on how to talk to one another with our bodies, with *and* without words. It is a skill that can be learned if you are open to learning it. But you have to want to be there with every part of your being, not just the conscious part, and you have to be willing to be open and vulnerable. Not many of us are really willing to be that visible, that exposed. Anna Marti puts it like this:

The most exciting erotic partner is one who is totally wired into it themselves and is having a really good time. They're probably having a good time regardless of who is going to be there. The erotic experience is really about having every cell in my body engaged.

Women are traditionally the givers and that is what we do: we give ourselves away, not in the sense of making ourselves vulnerable but in the sense of giving up our innate inner being. We give up our own needs in favor of our lover's.

"Giving" in this sense means prioritizing someone else's needs and feelings over our own, and many of us have specifically been taught that our needs are not as important as those of others. But it is a lie. We cannot be complete human beings if we do not pay attention to our own feelings. Feelings are what inform us of our needs, of what it is we should and should not do, of why we are here being human. Our feelings will guide us on the paths we must follow throughout our lives. Healthy sexual relationships are about balance, not sacrifice, about sharing, not withholding.

It Hurts So Good

There are many ways to have sex, many levels of passion, and many ways we can act out that passion. Having a skilled person make love to you slowly and gently, with the physical energy never building to a high crescendo, might be all you want. There are probably times when any of us might want only that, and there are other times when we want something quite different.

I've had nasty bad-ass sex with people I know very well and am very close to, and I've had very loving sex with people I hardly knew. Sometimes you just gotta do bad-ass sex.

These labels — bad-ass sex and lovemaking — are descriptive, and also misleading, since bad-ass sex can be about love just as much as lovemaking is. I'm going to label them **hard sex** and **soft sex**. Soft sex is what most women are expected to want. Many men are trying to be more sensitive, softer, and more gentle sexually. They are sweet and loving, they are very respectful, and they are trying to give women what they think we want. Soft sex, especially if it's done as a consciously tantric type of practice, may involve a very intense psychic experience, but it rarely involves a lot of physical exercise. It's often about transforming the physical sensations into a more emotional or spiritual realm.

I work at prolonging the stage just before orgasm and I often have to stop moving to stop myself coming. I try to equalize the energy throughout my body. Sometimes I feel like I'm coming through my skin. Depending on how intense and trusting we feel with each other, we become like light, and we move in and out of that place. Our spirits do an in/out merging thing, so we feel like one body with four arms and legs.

Hard sex is more about giving free reign to the physical manifestations of passion, and to the less acceptable feelings that come up for some of us during sexual play. It may be hard and fast and energetic, it may be slow, intense, and filled with suspense, and it may even be perceived as violent.

I like the interplay between reverence and nasty, sexually confrontational behavior. I crave that exchange and tension.

This sort of exchange might include teasing, bondage, role playing, voyeurism and exhibitionism, dominance and submission, spanking, or other forms of physical contact that would generally be experienced as painful or unpleasant in other circumstances; or it might include fantasies about such activities. And it might not include any of the above, but it will certainly include a level of physical passion that creates and is created by intense energy. In this state of arousal, the physical experience changes, and what would normally be uncomfortable can become profoundly erotic.

Under no circumstances whatsoever do I recommend any kind of sex during which either partner is not being fully respected. However, some women (and some men) need to have sex that is not always soft. Donna sums this up:

My partner is very in tune with me physically and psychically. And his approach to sex is a form of communication; from the beginning we've related physically. He's extremely intuitive. He also asks questions and then understands what I want immediately. But there's something more than that — he's not afraid of hurting me, he knows he's not hurting me, so he's much more . . . I don't know the word. Maybe it's that there is more freedom and abandon with him. With other partners there have always been more constraints.

These constraints are about sublimating the physical. As in so many areas of our lives, the prevailing mode of relating to someone of the opposite sex is clearly reflected in the sex act itself: the man is assumed to be the dominant one, the one who takes charge, who "runs the act," and in the process of asserting his desire and his needs, he must be careful not to hurt the woman he is with. It is rarely assumed that the man is in any danger of being hurt by his female partner. It is assumed that he is bigger, rougher, and stronger, and so is his desire. In reality, when a woman allows her body's passion and desire to take over, it becomes less likely for her to get physically hurt. You have two bodies dancing together; where one moves forward, the other gives way.

Michael, who is clearly used to being with passionate women, expresses this very well:

When I'm inside her, most often I just try to let my body accommodate her, the grinding and thrusting against me, picking up her rhythm or her shifting position to provide the kind of contact she needs. I make myself an instrument of her pleasure and I really enjoy being used that way. When I'm going down on her the force of her thrusting against my face can occasionally be quite uncomfortable, but I'm so caught up in her experience that I really don't mind. It's very exciting and I love the ride.

It is unfortunate, not just that men are usually running the act and that women tend to be alarmed by intense physical passion, but that so many people think that this is the way it should be. There are too many "shoulds" surrounding our sexual desires. Some women desire sex just as much as the most macho man, and some men desire sex as little (which may be not at all) as the most asexual woman. Women can orgasm just as quickly as men, given the right stimulation. Under the right circumstances, a woman's sexual appetite can be just as large or larger than a man's. Sexual stereotyping limits us all.

Fears versus Passion

When a couple come together unafraid of one another, and they refuse to be limited by false stereotyping or the fear of experiencing pain, then opportunities for unlimited passion will open up for them. We are all, men and women, responsible for creating these opportunities by letting go of restrictive, outmoded assumptions. Whether you are a man whose ego is tied up in a certain kind of sexual performance, or a woman who is afraid of taking the initiative, you must open up to new ways of being, and be willing to take risks if you hope to experience your full potential for ecstasy.

Now is the time for women to reclaim the power, intensity, and varieties of our orgasms — that knowledge has been lost and repressed — but to do so we must be willing to be animalistic, experimental, uninhibited, and uncontrollable. —Annie Sprinkle

We may be afraid that if we let go of the constraints we have adopted so that we will appear civilized, then we will not know when to stop, and we are terrified of what we might become if we don't stay in control. Ironically, these fears are the more intense *because* we deny them. If and when we let them out, they generally become quite manageable. The fantasies of being raped or of hurting someone that haunt so many women turn out to be just that — fantasies of being powerless or powerful. They reflect absolutely nothing about the reality of our everyday lives. Rather, they reflect an internal need to experiment with some aspect of ourselves that wants expression. Think of it as your "shadow" side. It is unavoidably a part of who you are, but not a part that is appropriate for public consumption. And that's fine, because there is no reason why you shouldn't be able to find a safe place to act it out in private with a trusted partner. And there is every possibility you can have a lot of fun with it.

When I was twenty-two, I was making out with my lover on her couch when she jumped up and said, "Stay right there, I'll be back in a minute!" She came back with a rope and said, "Look! Put your hands up here." Then she tied my hands and feet and made love to me. I came and came and came . . .

Talk to your partner about your fantasies, or the feelings that sometimes surge up when you let yourself express your desire. Discuss the possibility of acting them out. You could even plan a scenario and assign yourselves roles to play. See what happens. You may very well find that verbalizing the fantasy or the feeling is all you really needed. You may also discover that you enjoy playing out your fantasies. I think of this kind of play as an erotic party game or an adult form of cops and robbers. I clearly remember getting the same kind of excited high out of cops and robbers when I was a child as I do now, as an adult, from sexual games.

This is one fantasy that a friend of mine has had since she was a little girl. It's not one that should be acted out! But you could base some interesting games on it.

I imagined that I had a guy tied up and I was stimulating him sexually. He was getting really excited, but we both knew that at the moment when he came I would kill him. He always got to the point where he couldn't control himself any more . . .

With hard sex, as with soft sex, the key is **consensuality**, which means that each partner commits to full participation.

A sexual exchange may look sweet and loving, but if it is not fully consensual, it is not loving. On the other hand, a sexual act may look violent and dangerous, but if it is fully consensual, then it is a loving exchange. All is not that it appears to be on the surface. While I certainly do not need hard sex all the time, it is an essential part of my repertoire. I see it as a valuable forum for many women and men, one where we can safely express a level of passion that may have no other harmless outlets.

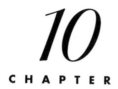

CHAPTER

From the Point of View of the Penis

It makes sense that there are hormonal differences and evolutionary differences between men and women, but that doesn't mean that men need to go around being gorillas. On the other hand, some men have really given up their sexuality to be acceptable as feminists. My politics and my sexuality are important to me, I'm not giving up either one. — David Steinberg

My husband, "impotent" for over twenty years, makes love like a woman, bless him, using fingers and tongue.

It may sound contradictory, but in a male-dominated society, with such an imbalance of masculine and feminine energies, men are bound to suffer, though in different ways from women. The male role has been as limiting for men as the female role has been for women, and men are finally beginning to understand this. Here in the United States we are seeing a swing towards the more "masculine" virtues of independence, strength, practicality, and assertiveness in women. We are also beginning to see men getting in touch with their feelings, moving away from the "rational" intellect, and showing less investment in being in charge. Hopefully we all get to meet in the middle at some point.

Popular Mythology

There is a widespread assumption, fostered by religious, cultural, and political influences, that men and women are made for each other, fitting together seamlessly with no rough edges and no effort. In reality, men and women having sex together are as likely to encounter problems as two women or two men. Some issues are due to genuine differences between the genders, but most are the result of social pressures.

Let's look at some of the assumed differences and see how real they actually are:

- sex is easy for men and men come from less specific stimulation; women need very specific stimulation in order to come;
- men are quick to get excited and quick to orgasm; women are slower to get excited and slower to orgasm;
- men come easily from intercourse; women often don't come at all from intercourse;
- once a man has come it's over for him; women want to carry on;
- men need sex more than women do;
- women need to feel a heart connection (trust) with their lovers; men don't need to feel an emotional connection.

Is Sex Easier for Men?

I am sure sex is easy for some men, as it is for some women, but just because men don't spend prodigious amounts of time and money putting on makeup, dressing, or having their hair done doesn't mean they don't get anxious about sexual encounters. In fact, the pressure on men to "perform" (terrible word) is more acute, since men are not supposed to be anxious. And yet they can't pretend: they either have an erection or they don't. Although there is no reason why a man and a woman shouldn't have a great time together sexually without his ever having an erection, the prevailing social view is that good sex depends on a man getting hard and staying hard. Dr. Joan Spiegel says:

There are many more men who feel insecure about their sexuality than you would think, because it's a real burden for men to be "a real man" who can have an erection any time. Most men feel, "Oh, I can't measure up!" The longer I've been a sex therapist the more I've come to appreciate the man's problem as well as the woman's.

The very word "performance" indicates they are doing it to show someone else, presumably an audience, what they can do. Indeed, that is what sex has been for many men: a demonstration of their virility, intended to impress. But an audience that is observing a performance gets to applaud or boo. Although few people verbalize it, the reality of this makes men incredibly vulnerable. One response to this feeling of vulnerability is the inability to perform:

Almost every time I am with a new person, I can't get an erection.

As we have seen in previous chapters, many women are able to orgasm from nonspecific and sometimes even nonphysical stimulation. Yet within the context of partnered sex, perhaps especially with a man, it seems that the woman is sometimes very particular, and it may be hard for her partner to "get it right." This may have practical causes. Although there are certain subtleties in pleasuring a man, one can often get away with very little skill, and the man usually has no problem being in control, setting the pace, pleasuring himself through intercourse.

Women often have a better idea of what is going to get a man aroused than most guys do about how to arouse a woman. It's not the female nature, that women get less aroused than men, it's that the sex that is happening is guy sex. — David Steinberg

A woman may be much less willing to direct the action, and more likely to lie back and have it done to her, hoping it's done right. Moreover, female genitalia are also less physically accessible. You get your finger on a clitoris and you have three potential problems: slipping off the particular spot (for some women the sensation must be in a very specific place), losing the right rhythm, and doing it too roughly or too softly. It is certainly a learnable skill, but not one that occurs automatically, and men are offered few opportunities to train. Somehow, they are just expected to know.

Women may not come easily because they need to feel emotional safety with their partner before they can let go into orgasm. This is a need that many men also feel. David Steinberg has found that anorgasmia is surprisingly common in men; that some men, like some women, find it easy to climax when they are alone, but have difficulty in the presence of a partner. In other words, they experience sex as something that makes them feel vulnerable, and they have to feel trust with their partner in order to orgasm. David himself stressed that it was important for him to trust his partner:

I've always experienced greater performance anxiety with women I don't know well; emotional and psychic safety are big issues for me. I think this is true for a lot of men. If I'm with someone I trust, I don't have to adopt a persona, I can just be who I am and feel what I feel. I think men tend to underestimate their need for safety. Lots of times they don't feel safe with their partners.

Are Men Aroused More Quickly?

As for speed, men and women have been known to masturbate to orgasm at exactly the same rates. I think I am probably fairly representative of the average woman. Depending on how aroused I am to start with, I can reach orgasm in a matter of seconds with a vibrator. With my hand I can sometimes reach orgasm in two or three minutes, although it takes me about fifteen minutes on average. With a skilled lover, it is the same. I have only had one lover who can make me come as quickly with her hand as I can make myself come with mine. I don't know what makes her so good — she just senses the right rhythm. So it certainly is possible for women to have quickies.

However, with male-female couples, it often seems as though men become aroused more quickly and want to get it over with, whereas women want to linger. The question is, if it feels good to men, why don't they also want to prolong the experience, rather than just "fuck and come"? Why do they want to get it over with? A quickie has its place, but if you never do anything else, you can't really be experiencing the pleasure on all levels.

Men are kind of overwhelmed by how quickly they get turned on, and so just want to do it right away. What seems to improve sex the most for men is if they can become less focused on orgasm, and become less anxious about whether they will momentarily lose their erection, and focus instead on the sensation of their whole body and try to put off having an orgasm as long as possible so that the tension can build; then they'll have much better orgasms. Men have such a tendency to be goal-oriented, and for the goal to be: "How fast I can make her come and how fast I can make myself come." It's the difference between fast food and fine dining. For most women the only true sexual fast food is a vibrator. — NightOwl

Is Intercourse Better for Men Than for Women?

Intercourse is simply more suited to direct and expedient stimulation of a penis than a clitoris. Although this a biological fact, there is absolutely no necessity for this to be a problem unless all a couple does is engage in intercourse. And if that is the case, then that, in itself, is a problem. Men and women can get fixated on intercourse to the exclusion of other activities. In reality, there are many ways of getting sexual pleasure. In these days of artificial insemination, intercourse is not even required for procreation. As David Steinberg says:

There's something special about intercourse, but it's not the be-

all and end-all of sex. I have a pretty diffuse sensual take on being sexual anyway. Sex is a whole body thing. G spot stimulation is about hands, for instance.

I do not mean to belittle intercourse. It can be enormously enjoyable for both men and women. But the importance that is placed on it, to the exclusion of all else, can be an impediment to sexual pleasure. And the importance placed on a man being able to get an erection is equally damaging. It is a lot like the pressure put on women to have orgasms. Just as a woman cannot force herself to have an orgasm, a man cannot force himself to have an erection. There is a similar social stigma attached to both of them. And it is that social stigma that creates so much pain for the individuals who see themselves as having failed.

Are Men Still Focused on Getting It Over With?

If a man is focused purely on his own pleasure, and he considers that pleasure to be his orgasm, then he will probably achieve it very quickly. But this indicates to me that he doesn't really want be there with the woman.

Most of the men who answered my questionnaire claimed they normally spent an hour or more making love. But the time from the insertion of the penis to removal of the penis varied from five minutes to an hour. Men can learn to take much longer if they want to, and their partners can assist them in this. If a man really wants to delay his climax then he can refrain from indulging in activities that will bring him

to orgasm until he decides the time is right. Learning to pleasure their female lovers so that they come more quickly is
another option. And men can also learn to continue with
lovemaking after their first orgasm. According to Alan and
Donna Brauer, exponents of Extended Sexual Orgasm, along
with many tantric teachers, men can develop the ability to
have multiple orgasms, non-ejaculatory orgasms, and
extended orgasms.

Do Men Need Sex More Than Women Do?

I think this is one of our most persistent myths, and what
truth it holds exists only because we have been thoroughly
indoctrinated in its perpetuation.

*The culture gives reinforcement to men feeling sexual desire for
its own sake, and women are discouraged from that, and told
to put it in the context of a relationship.* — David Steinberg

Sexy women have been belittled, reviled, ostracized,
raped, and murdered for centuries. Many people still believe
that if a woman walks down the street on a dark night wearing a miniskirt, she is asking to be raped and she deserves it
if it happens. Charges of rape were routinely dropped if it
could be proven that the victim had been promiscuous or
been thought to be promiscuous at any point in her life. It is
still standard practice in rape cases to defame the woman's
character.

Moreover, in the conventional sexual relationship dynamic,
there is less at stake for the man than for the woman. He is

very much less likely to be dependent on his lover economically, so he has no fear of losing his income if he has sex outside his marriage. He has no fear of getting pregnant, and is probably less likely to get emotionally attached. He is far less susceptible to contracting HIV from an infected woman than a woman is from an infected man. And his promiscuity is "proving" his virility, whereas a woman with many lovers is proving her "bad girl" status. On top of all of this very powerful conditioning, we have been encouraged to have sex in ways that don't tend to get women aroused, thus they may well not want to have conventional sex, and this could be interpreted as not wanting to have sex at all.

Do Men Need a Heart Connection Less Than Women Do?

We've been taught to believe that women are more emotional and men are less so, and we reinforce this training by acting out these stereotypes:

What women learn in high school is true: men give love to get sex and women give sex to get love.

But we don't have to. Wolfgang Ronnefeldt, who is now fifty-six, says:

The most important thing for me is the heart connection, and the rest follows, but it's taken years of refinement to get to this point.

Wolfgang's need is reflected by a number of other men:

My favorite part of sex is being accepted and desired, to fill an intimate and very personal need or desire.

When I was younger it was sex for the sake of sex. With my wife it's being with her, holding her, and knowing that we are both about to have a really good time.

What I enjoy most is the closeness, the kissing, and touching.

Having an emotional connection with a woman, or simply feeling strong emotions, is frightening for many men. If they don't know how to be emotionally present, they may react to strong feelings by cutting themselves off from them as quickly as possible. I have a theory that this is why so many men want to roll straight over and go to sleep right after sex; feeling the intense connection that comes from sharing one's body so intimately is alarming to them.

The belief that men are less vulnerable, less in need of nurturing, and less prone to intense emotion than women is another classic myth, and it is one that has been, if anything, more damaging to men than to women, because they have tried to live up to it. The good news is that men are becoming dissatisfied with sex that is divorced from emotion.

The best part of sex is to see the love and passion in her eyes, to know she feels the love I offer her.

Sexual Dysfunction and the Need for Nurturing

Our society does not encourage men to ask for nurturing. Look at the following stereotypes:

- women want to be taken care of;
- men owe it to women to take care of them;
- women are basically more emotionally fragile than men;

- men can take care of their own needs, and anyway they don't have as many needs as women;
- men are insensitive, women are overly sensitive;
- men are more rational and less emotional than women;
- men are more powerful, more efficient, and more capable than women;
- men are more dominant, and women tend to be submissive;
- men's egos are more fragile than women's, and women need to be careful not to criticize their men;
- women who are motherly can't also be sexy.

These stereotypes prevent men and women from getting their needs met. Bill says:

I really suspect that most male bragging about sex is a far cry from reality. I think most men are looking for nurturing and comfort, and they don't know how to ask for it. They don't really know how to communicate with their wives at all.

Such damaging stereotypes, and the impossibility of living up to them, seem to be at the root of many of the sexual dysfunctions that men suffer from, including anorgasmia, premature ejaculation, loss of desire, and lack of erection.

One of the men who was so helpful to me when I began writing this chapter was Dave from the Liberated Christians group:

Being unable to maintain an erection happens a lot to us men over forty. It's perfectly normal, but many men I know are concerned. My first failure experience was on my fortieth birthday when my partner had a wonderful sensual evening with me.

She was wonderful but I was dead. It is very frustrating, but few are willing to discuss it.

He goes on to say that although he gets anxious about his ability to maintain an erection, he doesn't feel like a failure, and he finds plenty of other ways to please a woman, such as G spot stimulation with his fingers. There is no doubt that Dave's sense of security is unusual. Eddy fully acknowledges that his self-image is tied up in getting and maintaining an erection:

If my erection isn't strong enough that the woman can come from intercourse, I would normally resort to using my hand, but it is still a blow to my self-esteem if her orgasm isn't from my penis.

Men who have small penises, ejaculate prematurely, or lose erections may all be suffering from deep feelings of anxiety around sex. But if they could get past their sense of inadequacy, they might find themselves at an advantage, because they must learn to use their hands and their tongues. People who are orally and manually skillful, who can communicate and listen, and who aren't held back by socially endorsed inhibitions, are people who make great lovers. And if she wants a big hard penis — there are always dildoes. In other words, if women and men could get over their ideas about the way things ought to be, all sorts of problems would simply disappear.

Perhaps men are not biologically designed to remain virile all their lives. But I think lack of erection, more than any of the other problems listed previously, is a result of changing status in a changing world. The erect penis is the symbol of a kind of manhood to which many men no longer wish to subscribe, or are no longer able to participate in. It used to be that men used their sexuality to establish dominance over women, and men who no longer wish to do this may be withholding their sexual power, consciously or unconsciously. They haven't found a nonoppressive way of giving their sexual power full reign. In her book, *Hands of Light* (Bantam Books, 1988), Barbara Brennan says that withholding sexual power creates a block in the second chakra, which will result in premature ejaculation or inability to achieve an erection.

Lack of erection doesn't necessarily mean a lack of desire. The sexual feelings may be as strong as ever. But men *are* also losing desire. Dr. Joan Spiegel treats as many couples in which the man has lost desire, as she does couples where the woman has lost desire. Loss of desire in women is often a result of withholding feelings, and I suspect the same is true of men. Because of the troubling feelings which arise whenever sexual desire arises, sexual desire must be repressed to keep the feelings buried. More men are experiencing less desire because they are finding themselves unable to bury their feelings any longer.

Emotional Baggage

Some men are having hotter sex outside marriage than in it. Eddy has trouble maintaining an erection with his wife if he is at all upset with her, yet with other women he has to battle to lose it. Statistics from a number of different studies show that many men are having extramarital affairs. I believe it's possible to have a heart connection with someone whom you barely know, and certainly with more than one lover at a time, so I don't think that men are necessarily trying to avoid intimacy by having sex with someone they don't know well.

The prevailing view is that it is familiarity that dulls passion. However, I believe that it is withholding emotion that dulls passion; failing to deal with the problems and differences that inevitably arise in any long-term relationship. I am not sure how a relationship that is free from emotional baggage might unfold, because so few people deal with their emotions cleanly. However, I am sure men are having hotter sex with women they don't have a lot of emotional baggage with. If men in long-term relationships want to continue to have great sex and maintain their erections, they must learn to deal with their repressed or unresolved feelings on a daily basis so that they don't accumulate a backlog of resentment and confusion.

When I've been upset with my wife and we've had an argument, I have to struggle to obtain an erection.

I once lost an erection for no apparent reason, but I was thinking of an argument we'd had earlier in the day.

In a short-term relationship, a man can maintain his facade. In a long-term relationship, real weaknesses and failings, which are only part of being human, after all, are bound to show through. Men are in a kind of no-man's land, where they are no longer infallible he-men, but they still haven't come to terms with being vulnerable human beings.

The New Focus: The Woman's Pleasure

*If one is focused on what one is doing to someone else, there
is a high probability that one is less fully present in one's own
experience, one's own body sensations. Men with erection dysfunction or premature ejaculation, especially erection dysfunction, often haven't been in their bodies for quite a long time.*
— Anna Marti

The changing focus of sex still leaves the man in charge. It
is now his responsibility to make sure the woman comes.
Being more concerned about pleasing his partner than about
having a good time together can be a way for him to take the
focus off his own feelings. But the result is that he isn't really
in his body.

He is not coming from a place within his body that knows
what's right and feels good; he is coming from an intellectual
place that says, "Women have a hard time having orgasms
and it's really easy for me to have one, so I'm going to put
my pleasure aside and make sure she has a really good time;
after all, that will be fulfilling for me in itself, and it will
prove I'm not a macho jerk." The focus on what makes a
man a man has shifted from how many times a day he can
get an erection, and how big that erection is, to how many
times a day he can bring his wife to orgasm.

The Durex survey corroborates this shift in focus. It reports
that 45 percent of American men are more concerned about
their partner's enjoyment than their own, compared to 32
percent of women. The questionnaire that I distributed to
men reflected the same information. I asked if men saw it as
their responsibility to give their partner an orgasm:

I feel it's my responsibility to engage in activities that are pleasing enough that my partner will be comfortable and relaxed enough to have an orgasm. It is an objective for me that she have an orgasm.

If giving her an orgasm is part of pleasing her, then I feel it's my responsibility to attempt to give her an orgasm.

Absolutely, I feel it's my responsibility to give her an orgasm.

I try to keep going until my partner has an orgasm.

I like to be able to please the woman I am with and make it an experience they will want to repeat and have pleasant memories of. If I somehow fail at this goal I would feel disappointed.

Several men stressed that the pleasure they got from their partner's pleasure was very intense, and sometimes their own need to orgasm was secondary.

The joy of watching her pleasure, her body trembling, her soft moans, is almost unbelievable. It is a greater joy than my own orgasm.

Women's orgasms are my greatest source of pleasure in love-making.

I like women to be able to enjoy their experience with me — that gives me as much or more pleasure than my own orgasm.

When she is coming I reach a level of arousal that can't be matched any other way.

It is wonderful that men are no longer jumping on top, pumping away until they're done, and then falling asleep. But if this means they are absenting themselves from their own bodies in order to be there for their partners, the change must continue. Men are still the doers, and women are the receivers; men are just trying to do better. They have exchanged one form of sexual prowess for another. There is a two-way street that has to be traveled, where men step back, women step forward, and they meet in the middle.

It has been suggested that men might look to lesbians for information about how to please women, and the average lesbian certainly knows much more about women's sexual pleasure than the average heterosexual man. But if what men want is to learn more about their *own* sexuality, which would be perfectly appropriate, they might look to gay men. The average gay man knows more about men's sexual pleasure than the average heterosexual woman. Men need to redefine their roles as sexual beings, and the gay male community might have something to offer.

To be fair, it is as much a woman's responsibility to take charge as it is a man's to surrender. And there may be just as many women who are not stepping forward as there are men who are not stepping back. It is so much easier for women to bad-mouth men than to take the risk of assuming responsibility for their own lives.

Do Men Know When We're Faking It?

According to the NHSLS survey of sexual practices, only 29 percent of women come regularly with a partner, but men think that 44 percent of their female partners come regularly. Does this mean that 15 percent of the time women are convincingly faking it? I admit I felt a bit doubtful about a couple of the questionnaires. A few men claimed that they had been with more than thirty women (in one case, fifty), all of whom had had orgasms, every time! Some men claimed that all their lovers came just from intercourse! In my opinion, either some of those women were faking it, or else their men assumed they were having orgasms because they appeared to be enjoying themselves.

In spite of the delightful scene in *When Harry Met Sally*, when Meg Ryan's character convincingly fakes an orgasm in a restaurant, most men are sure they would know when a woman is faking it. Let me debunk this myth for once and for all: it is easy for a woman to consciously contract her vaginal muscles. If she has any acting skills at all, and any real desire to con her partner, that person, male or female, would very likely walk away from the encounter thinking she had an orgasm. If her partner does get suspicious, it may be because she wants him or her to notice that something is not right.

It is hardly surprising that most men really didn't like knowing or suspecting that a woman was faking it:

One woman I was with claimed to have these astronomical orgasms, but I was pretty inexperienced at the time and when I think back to some of the things I did, I just shake my head. I doubt they really happened.

One of my exes told me she had faked orgasm with me. I felt like it was too bad we couldn't have really tried together to bring her to that experience.

I have suspected a woman of faking orgasm because of obvious theatrics or because her physical state suggested that she was not actually in an advanced state of passion. I cannot bear the thought of a woman giving herself to me without finding pleasure in the intimacy of lovemaking. I would much rather that she found pleasure than I. After loving a woman who I felt was faking it, I tend to feel inadequate I suppose. It leaves me empty inside.

Once I suspected one of my lovers of faking orgasm so I simply asked her and after trying to lie she finally admitted it was unusual for her to achieve orgasm, but she still enjoyed the intimacy.

I felt as if I had been lied to. Loving is not a game, it is of the heart, of the soul, of the tenderness that wells up inside just from the nearness of your lover. To have her fake an orgasm is hurtful.

After a long period of lovemaking, one girlfriend seemed to come really fast and then seemed to want it to be over, as if she thought I was still doing it waiting for her to come. I felt bad only because I wanted her to know I was being sexual with her because I enjoyed it.

Many of us fake it because we're not enjoying ourselves. I remember lying there (years ago) with a man heaving to and fro on top of me, thinking, how can I gracefully end this as soon as possible? The fact that he was enjoying it when I wasn't made me feel more alienated, as though he was using my body only for his pleasure. And it never entered my head that he might not be enjoying himself. Like many women, I thought I was the only person in the world who didn't enjoy sex. And I thought all men enjoyed it *all* the time.

But we also fake it because we are ashamed of not being able to come, or of being thought frigid; because we are afraid of talking about what we need, and ashamed of having to ask. If they choose to do so, men can help women to feel easier about acknowledging what is really going on.

Not all men seem to mind a woman faking orgasm:

My wife has faked it more than once. I found out by asking her. Frankly, it's flattering to me — it tells me that she wants me to feel as if I had done a good job.

I think he could have been flattered if she had talked to him about it, instead of faking it. He could have appreciated that she respected him enough to believe that he would be more concerned about their relationship than about his ego. And I would think that he would have respected her for being truthful with him. But then, my idea of intimacy does not include being intimate with someone who thinks it's okay to lie to me, or for me to lie to them.

The bottom line is that faking anything is an attempt to live up to a model that isn't working for you, and if you acknowledge that it isn't working, you might be able to do something that does. As Eric says:

I hate it that she wasn't honest with me. If we could have talked about it maybe she would have had those orgasms for real.

Sharing Roles and Challenging Established Patterns

Moving beyond the time-honored patterns of heterosexuality may require constant effort and vigilance. Victoria, who had relationships with women for years and is now with a man, spells out what it takes to maintain balance in her relationship with her husband:

There is an inherent power imbalance in heterosexual relation-ships and it cannot be changed unilaterally. It requires men and women both being committed to changing it for themselves. One crucially important aspect of my relationship with my partner is that if something happens that resembles a male point of privilege, I'm able to point this out, and he's able to hear it, take it seriously, and redress the problem. Also, I'm able to make casual references to the realities without him get-ting all defensive, and moreover, he himself makes casual ref-erences to the realities, which lets me know on an ongoing basis that he gets it. It requires a huge commitment, because there's not much support in the culture for such a relationship. It's far too easy to let a little thing slide here and there until there's no getting back. But such relationships are the only hope, I think, for women and men to find happiness together. In such relationships, honesty is finally possible, and honesty is a prerequisite to intimacy.

If a woman questions the power dynamic in her marriage without the support of her husband, she is sure to meet with enormous resistance from him if his self-image is based on the assumption that he is the dominant member of the part-nership, or that the world sees him that way. Even if he admits that he would occasionally like to drop the burden of responsibility, it is not an easy thing to do when his self-esteem is based on an appearance of shouldering this burden effortlessly.

Men who do want to challenge the status quo face a long, lonely road. Other men may see them as enemies, as traitors who have defected. A man who is willing to make himself vulnerable and refuses to comply with established social pat-terns is going to have trouble finding support. And yet it is essential that men begin to acknowledge that they have feel-ings and needs that are just as powerful as ours; that they cannot live up to the standard of macho manhood; and that we don't necessarily want them to.

Even if a man makes a conscious decision to challenge conventional gender roles, there will be occasions when he is uncomfortable with his choice. When I asked Eric how he would feel about his female lover strapping on a dildo and penetrating him anally, he answered, very honestly, that he would find it unnerving and degrading:

I'm really not sure why. It's actually quite the double standard because I've done anal sex on women before. Maybe it's a power/security thing: the woman, supposedly weaker, on the ramming end?

I asked him if he would feel the same way if it were a man performing anal sex on him and he said he didn't think so. I believe Eric was being honest. He was not saying he thought women to be the weaker sex, but rather acknowledged that he might be affected by the fact that it was an established belief in this society until very recently. Eric is certainly not a macho jerk. As a matter of fact, I was very impressed when I received his questionnaire response. What came through was a man who really cares about women, really wants to do his best for them in bed, goes to great lengths to find out what they want, and prefers women who have claimed their power.

It may be that Eric is one of those people who just doesn't want to be on the bottom, meaning it doesn't turn him on to be the submissive partner in an erotic exchange. But he does mention that his present partner is quite submissive and he doesn't like that. Several other men mentioned that they would like their female partners to be more assertive. Dan (who's never experienced anal penetration) says he is very attracted to the idea of anal sex:

I get very aroused when I fantasize about getting fucked by a woman with a great big strap-on dildo. Wow! Hot, hot, hot! If my wife would go for it, I'd love to slip into a submissive role occasionally. Unfortunately she has trouble with a domineering role.

Alas, Dan is unusual. Most heterosexual men are terrified of receiving anal sex — they really don't want to want it. There is a missed potential here. I have to agree with Carol Queen when she says:

Anally erotic men have already broken a taboo and taken one step toward creating the sexuality they really want, not the one society told them was theirs to embrace. (Real Live Nude Girl, Cleis Press)

I would not choose to be a man in this world — they appear to have plenty of benefits on the surface, but it is difficult for them to challenge the status quo; to acknowledge, and therefore overcome, their fears. Women today have begun to come into their power in all its depth and glory, and we have developed networks of support in many different arenas. We are engaged in a massive healing process that is both unifying and liberating. Most men are still committed to the external trappings of power by which they define themselves. This means they remain committed to leading lives that are, at worst, shallow and destructive, and at best, unfulfilling.

The Male Experience of Female Orgasm

Before ending this chapter, I want to offer some comments from men that illustrate what they experience physically when a woman comes.

I often feel a chemical change in vaginal fluid during her orgasm. It seems to sensitize me and encourage my own orgasm.

I physically feel a sort of second-hand orgasm when the woman I am with comes. If my penis is inside her I feel the contractions of her muscles.

With some women there is no noticeable physical difference when they are coming, and other women have vaginal contractions so powerful that it goes well past my pain threshold. There are lots of women in between where the contractions and the gyrations of her ecstasy are a source of great pleasure that often make it difficult not to come myself.

I mostly feel muscle contractions when she comes; sometimes I sense an angle change and a change in tightness. Sometimes there is a feeling of tightening but mostly it is a feeling of some relaxation and softening to some extent.

I enjoy having her reach orgasm through oral stimulation the most. She ejaculates a lot and I really enjoy the taste and feel of her flowing out on my face and in my mouth. I experience an intense emotional rush, similar to a peaking sensation just prior to orgasm.

I see stars. I love it when she crushes my head with her legs.

I'm usually attempting to breathe while she cuts off the circulation to my head with her arms!

Whether because younger women today are more likely to "expose" themselves to, or be more open with men, or whether it is the men who are changing, the questionnaires from younger men tended to reflect more understanding of women than those from older men. Here are four comments, from men aged (respectively) sixteen, twenty-seven, nineteen, and twenty-one, that illustrate a level of wisdom I certainly never encountered during the years I was sexually active with men.

There is no activity that commonly brings women to orgasm; it's the passion and intensity that does.

Women's orgasms are hard to predict: like a storm. I have to pay attention to body language in order to be relatively certain a woman is actually having one.

If sex was satisfying for me and not for her, it's time to get oral.

Masturbation is the key to women having orgasms. By masturbating, she finds out more about what works for her and what doesn't.

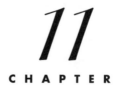

C H A P T E R

Penetration and the G Spot

My lover once penetrated me so deeply with her hand that I felt as though something I didn't know existed had exploded (pleasantly!)

Lubrication

ny chapter on penetration must start with a eulogy about the wonders of artificial lubrication. Even if you never engage in any kind of penetration, good lubrication and plenty of it will radically improve your sex life. In my experience, very few women produce enough natural lubrication to enjoy penetration or manual clitoral stimulation for long without some discomfort. Good lubrication will enormously enhance your enjoyment, enable you to carry on much longer, and considerably reduce the risk of getting vaginal or urinary tract infections. Older women tend to have less natural lubrication, but the quantity of natural lubrication we produce varies: some women get very creamy very quickly, while others produce little wetness even when they are very turned on. If you are one of the latter, you will want to use artificial lubrication whenever you engage in sexual activities, but even for those of you who get very wet, I would recommend having a bottle of lube on hand for all sexual play. There may be times when you want to prolong a session of lovemaking, but you start to get a little sore. On these occasions, the use of a lubricant can make the difference between a yeast infection, a bladder infection, and no infection at all. Some parts of our bodies, such as the anus, don't naturally produce lubrication. You *must* use artificial lubrication if you are going to be anally penetrated. Besides all that, lube has a very sensuous and silky feel to it.

Sex definitely felt very uncomfortable until I discovered lube — that made a big difference.

The most common kinds of artificial lubrication, made specifically for use during sex, are water-based, which means two things: they will wash out of the vagina easily, and they will not degrade condoms. Oil-based products — vegetable, mineral, or petroleum, which include Crisco, baby oil, Vaseline, and most massage oils — will degrade latex condoms or gloves.

One of the stupidest things I ever did was have sex with this guy when all we had to use for lube was olive oil. Believe me, olive oil destroys condoms.

Silicone-based lubes have just come on the market, and they don't degrade latex (although they do damage silicone dildoes). I have heard of women having allergic reactions to these. You need to find out what works for you; there are enough choices that you don't need to use anything you find irritating.

If you are not using latex condoms or gloves, of course you can use massage oil for lubrication, but I recommend not using anything that is mineral-based on any sensitive, or potentially tender, parts of your anatomy. Some women are allergic to mineral-based oils, and moreover, oils don't wash out of the vagina as readily as water-based lubes, and they tend to encourage the growth of bacteria.

Some lubes have a high level of glycerine in them and this makes them sweet, which may promote the growth of yeast cells. Some are foamy, some are smooth, some dry out more quickly than others, some are runnier, some are thicker. Some reconstitute when you add water (so beware of spills that dry out and appear harmless until you try to wash them away, and they turn into a slippery morass!), which means you can use them sparingly because you can add a few drops of water instead of lube when they start to dry out. KY Jelly, which is probably what your doctor uses when she examines you, comes in a tube rather than a bottle. It is perfectly adequate, but doesn't feel quite as silky as some other brands, and tastes worse than most, although none of them actually taste very good. Some contain nonoxynol-9, a chemical that kills the AIDS virus. But nonoxynol-9 is an irritant, and many women are allergic to it. I don't recommend it.

You don't need to go into a sex store to buy lube — there are a variety of products available at the pharmacy. If you'd like a wide selection, get a catalog from Good Vibrations or Blowfish.

Some people are allergic to latex. Condoms and gloves made from other substances, such as nitrile, are available. It may be the powder on the gloves that causes allergic reactions, or the type of lube on prelubed condoms. You can buy unlubed condoms at well-stocked pharmacies, but be sure to read the package. Unpowdered gloves are also available, although they may be harder to obtain.

The PC Muscle

If you are going to enjoy penetration, and have good orgasms, it is a good idea to have well-toned muscles in the pelvic area, and, in particular, a healthy pubococcygeal (PC) muscle. This is the sling of muscle that supports the sexual organs, and I believe it should be considered as integral to a woman's sexual make-up as the clitoris or the G spot. Just as different parts of the body work together to make us functional human beings, the different parts involved in sexual response work together to enable us to experience full sexual enjoyment. Chronic tension or weakness of the PC muscle can radically affect our sexual responses. Not surprisingly, women who are afraid of, or uptight about sex, may have a chronically tense or weak PC muscle. According to *The G Spot* (by Ladas, Whipple and Perry, first published in 1982 by Holt, Rinehart and Winston), a woman with a strong PC muscle is more likely to have orgasms, strong orgasms, multiple orgasms, and different kinds of orgasms. She may also produce more natural lubrication.

Having sex and orgasming are a workout for this muscle, but there are also specific exercises that you can do, called Kegels, which were originally developed by Dr. Arnold Kegel to help his patients with urinary problems. You can buy something called a Kegelciser, which looks like a tiny dumb-bell, that you insert into the vagina, and then practice holding it in there and making it move. You can also practice tightening and relaxing that muscle at other times. Try to isolate it from the muscles in your buttocks and your belly, because you may be failing to exercise the PC muscle if you don't. To check your progress, you can isolate the PC muscle by stopping the flow of urine in the middle of urination. However, you should not make this a regular practice or training method because the continual interruption of urine flow can increase the risk of urinary tract infection.

Once you've sorted out what the muscle feels like, you can do sets of exercises. A typical set would include: clench-ing slowly and then relaxing ten times; clenching as fast as you can ten times (flutters); and pushing outwardly ten times. Work up to doing thirty repetitions within each set, five times a day.

Some women find the sexual awareness that results from doing Kegels uncomfortable: you may not welcome an overt sensation of desire, when you are just trying to get on with your life. There you are sitting at your desk working away, when one of your co-workers comes over to discuss some-thing with you. You feel a flush of turn-on and your PC mus-cle contracts, grabbing your attention. It might be easier to be able to ignore your body. Once again, you have to decide your own priorities: how much time and energy are you will-ing to spend on sex? What if your sexual desire arises at a time when it's not "appropriate"?

Women who are uncomfortable with their sexual responses are going to cut off their awareness of the PC muscle, without even knowing what they are doing, because it is an effective way to cut off their awareness of their sexual responses. What if they find themselves responding to another woman, and have ambivalent or negative feelings about homosexuality and bisexuality? What if they want to be faithful to their husbands? What if they respond to images of bondage, and they believe this response is deviant? Deciding *not* to make a negative judgement about what turns you on is a necessary prerequisite for toning your PC muscle. As long as you are cutting yourself off from any muscular responses that your brain deems unacceptable, you are cutting your mind off from your body, and limiting the possibility of being a whole, healthy human being.

The advantages to a healthy PC muscle are not just sexual. A woman with a well-toned PC muscle is less likely to have bladder problems, she will probably have an easier time with childbirth, and she is far less likely to suffer from a prolapsed uterus. She may even find that her periods become more regular. Women who suffer from cystitis or vaginal infections may find Kegel exercises surprisingly beneficial. Severe cramps (menstrual or otherwise) and low back pain can sometimes be traced to an overly tense PC muscle.

I know of a few women who can come just by flexing their PC muscle. A number of women report that they are able to orgasm from vaginal penetration alone after doing Kegel exercises for several months. (Having an orgasm from vaginal penetration alone, without any direct stimulation of the clitoris, is something many women think they ought to be able to do, but rarely can.)

Having very strong muscles isn't necessarily preferable for your partner, as this quote from a man illustrates:

I had one partner who had the most incredibly strong vaginal muscles. She could induce pain without externally visible signs, not even a facial twitch or grimace. I have a very strong grip, and I cannot squeeze my penis hard enough to cause pain. She could — with her vagina. I had to ask her to be careful, which was difficult for her when she was in the middle of an orgasm.

However, a woman with a well-toned PC muscle, able both to relax it fully and to tighten it, is a woman who is sexually aware and responsive, no matter how she reaches orgasm.

I've learned to come through muscle control, with no direct physical stimulation at all. This basically involves doing Kegels, although I've found that mentally focusing on the area just inside my vagina and at the front helps a lot.

Note that it is as important to be able to relax it as it is to be able to tense it. You may have a very strong PC muscle, but if you are unable to relax it, then you will have problems, just as you would with any chronically tight muscle in your body.

Penetration Is Not Essential

Muscles sometimes become chronically tense for emotional or psychological reasons, and this is commonly the case with the PC muscle, perhaps because we have so much emotional and psychological baggage associated with sex. If a woman is afraid of penetration or intercourse (and there are many reasons why she might be), then fear will cause her to tense her PC muscle. Suddenly her vagina is smaller and tighter than it normally is, and intercourse will inevitably be painful. The medical term for this is vaginismus, and it is not uncommon. If this is a problem for you, then I urge you to seriously consider whether or not you want penetration at all. I know lesbians who have very satisfying sex who never or rarely receive penetration. There is no reason why the same shouldn't be true for heterosexual women, but there is societal pressure, and probably pressure from their lovers also, on heterosexual women to indulge in vaginal penetration.

As a teenager I had intercourse with lots of guys and it seemed like a real waste of time. The best sex I had in those days was when I refused to have intercourse with this one guy and he got me off with his fingers on my clitoris. That was great.

The best orgasm I ever had involved no penetration at all; it just came from this utterly animal desire. I was on top of her, we both had all our clothes on, and we were just rubbing our bodies on each other. Neither of us were doing anything to the other, no one was directing anything. The orgasm just exploded out of me. She came at the same moment.

Linda Valins, who suffers from vaginismus herself, has written a book on the subject, called *When a Woman's Body Says No to Sex*. This is an interesting book, but it is important to understand that women whose vaginas tighten up when they are about to be penetrated vaginally are not necessarily saying no to sex. I believe they are saying no to penetration

271

in particular. They are still able to have very enjoyable sex. Penetration is like the color pink, or riding horses, or anything else in life: some people just don't like it.

I sometimes like vaginal penetration, but only if I'm very turned on.

I have never felt the need for penetration during sex. It's not that I abhor it, but it does nothing for me. I don't get turned on by it. I don't feel anything much and so it happens only because my partner wants to do it. For orgasms I need my clitoris touched. The vagina can take it or leave it.

But Some of Us Really Love It!

Plenty of women, lesbians and heterosexuals (myself included), cannot imagine satisfying sex that doesn't involve penetration. It wasn't always this way for me, however; I spent at least five years during my twenties doing sex with little or no penetration before I began to really want it. What happened? I'd have to guess since there was no obvious cause or event: I believe it was simply that I began to relax around sexual issues, as a result of having good sex. As I began to enjoy it more and more, my PC muscle, with no conscious effort on my part, became very toned. As I worked on myself, I lost the psychological and emotional charge I once had around intercourse, and I became interested in penetration because I was getting more and more in touch with my own body.

Virginity: The Arduous Process of Losing It

Virginity is such a loaded concept in our society. It is supposed to be a major event when you lose it, and yet, I
haven't met many women whose experience was enjoyable.
Most of us have the same incredulous reaction to an event
that is supposed to be one of the most momentous of our
lives: You mean *that's it?!*

*It was the first time for both of us, and we were really inept. It
was one of those experiences that is funny in retrospect but
deeply mortifying at the time.*

*When I was seventeen, I met this guy who was much older. He
wouldn't have intercourse with me until I was eighteen. On my
eighteenth birthday he brought a condom out (I'd been asking
to have sex), and we did it. I didn't feel anything. It didn't hurt,
it was just boring. I lay there thinking, oh my god, this is it?! I
was so disappointed.*

*My first experiences with intercourse, as a teenager, didn't do
anything for me. The very first time I was with a guy my legs
went numb, I guess from him putting pressure on my thighs
while he was on top, and I thought that must be a vaginal
orgasm. I wasn't excited about it.*

*I'd decided it was time for me to lose my virginity and so I went
to bed with a guy. It was fairly clinical: quick, calculated, and a
little weird.*

*My boyfriend took me out to the country, we had a bottle of
champagne, and then did it on a blanket in a field. The setting
was beautiful, but the act was disappointing. I felt scared and
uncomfortable.*

*We were supposed to play this silly game where we were lead-
ing boys on and yet never allowing them to go the whole way.*

By the time I was fifteen, I was really bored with this absurd game — it just didn't make any sense to me — so I got myself a boyfriend and had intercourse with him. He told me I couldn't be a virgin because I wasn't scared enough.

My partner didn't believe I was a virgin. He thought I had lots of experience because of my enthusiasm and passion.

By contrast, Mary did enjoy her first experience with intercourse:

It felt great — a vibrator can't match how a big, hard cock feels!

Maybe what made it feel so good for Mary was that she had been masturbating, with penetration, for a number of years prior to her first time doing intercourse. Or perhaps her lover was simply more skilled.

But the crux of the matter is that most cultures place a ludicrous amount of importance on an act that is barely an event for most women, particularly as the hymen may well have been broken long before the moment of consensual penetration by a penis, either due to the use of tampons, or to molestation or masturbation. Fortunately, the social and biological concepts of virginity are finally beginning to change. Younger women may be reaping the benefits of these changes: greater access to information, a more caring attitude on the part of men, and more possibility that a woman will feel comfortable and proud in her sexual desire.

The bottom line with penetration is the same as the bottom line with sex: how important is it to you? If you decide it is important and now is the time when you want it, then you must choose a partner whom you trust to be caring and patient, and you must take steps to remove any sources of tension. If you worry about getting pregnant, then either use adequate birth control (your idea of adequate may not necessarily be the same as someone else's, and this is a situation where only *your* idea of adequate matters), or use something other than a penis for penetration: fingers and dildoes don't cause pregnancy.

Some men have very large penises, and they may have trouble finding women who can comfortably accommodate them. Like men with very small penises, they have to find other ways of making love. In a society where sexual play has been so overshadowed by the importance placed on intercourse, such men may be at an advantage. They have an incentive to learn how to satisfy a woman in other ways. (I heard of a man with a very large penis who would bring himself to orgasm by penetrating his lover's cleavage. This might work well for women with large and sensitive breasts. And then he gets to use his mouth and hands between her legs.)

I once had a partner who had a very small penis and he was the best lover I ever had. He'd had to learn to compensate.

Enjoying Penetration

If you are concerned about pain with intercourse then you may want to experiment on your own, putting your fingers, or something else, inside your vagina, so you are prepared for what it feels like. But, remember, you should be in control. If at any time you experience something you don't enjoy, you must be able to stop at once. Many men, especially inexperienced ones, attempt penetration too quickly, and if you aren't ready, then it won't feel good. It may take a woman a long time (hours, weeks, years) of experimentation before she is ready for intercourse. Are you unable to imagine asking your partner to stop in the middle of a sexual encounter? I have said it before and I will continue to repeat it: you must get into the habit of talking to your partner before, during, and after sex. Verbalize what feels good for you, asking him or her to slow down or speed up or change position to suit your desire. If he or she doesn't like taking direction from you, this is a serious problem that needs to be resolved before you carry on with a relationship.

Remember that if a woman is a virgin, she is likely to expect penetration to be painful, although, in fact, it isn't always so. Many women have lost their hymens by the time they embark on intercourse, and even if they haven't, the breaking of the hymen is an individual sensation. Some women experience a brief, sharp pain while others never notice a thing. The hymen can stretch quite considerably, so it is possible to experience penetration for quite a long time (months or even years) before it finally tears. Once it is fully torn, it should cause no further pain. But it doesn't always tear completely. Some women may find that a piece of it remains for years. If it is bothersome, it can be removed by a physician. Occasionally, a woman will have a very tough hymen that may give her trouble:

I had an unusually tough hymen and unsuccessfully attempted intercourse with one lover who, confronted with my inexorable

*virginity, became impotent. At twenty-one, I found this shatter-
ing. Was it my fault? It was particularly hard in light of early
molestation. When I did manage my first time it was with a
trusted (and undaunted) friend. It took us several awkward
tries. It hurt but it was also a relief.*

As with all sexual acts, trust is vital. It isn't just a matter of
trusting that your lover will respect your needs and take care
of you. You also have to trust your own body; you have to
believe that this is something your body wants, and is capable of enjoying. You have to believe that your body can open
up and relax and have a good time. Bad experiences with
penetration, childhood molestation, adult rape, clumsy partners, or even carelessly done vaginal exams may make a
woman's body reluctant to open up to the possibility of sexual pleasure.

*I was in an abusive relationship for a couple of years and for some
time after that I couldn't have orgasms, even with lovers who
were not at all abusive. It was like my feeling of self-trust had
been damaged, because I had allowed that abuse to happen to me.*

In the nineteenth century, it was quite normal for women
to experience intercourse as painful and unpleasant. A wife
did her duty by her husband; she did not expect to enjoy sex
with him and she would probably have worried about her
own morality if she had. Of course there were exceptions,
but it was quite an accepted cultural norm of the time.
Things have changed, and nowadays, a man is "supposed" to
take the time to make his wife happy in bed (and many truly
want to do so). Unfortunately, these Victorian ideas still lurk
in our subconscious, and there are women who expect inter-

course to be painful on a regular basis, not just the first time. And if they believe this then they will hold their bodies tightly to forestall the pain. A tight vagina does not generally welcome penetration, but there are plenty of things a couple can do that don't involve penetration, which will lead to the woman getting more and more turned on, so that at some point she will possibly feel the desire to have something inside her. Start with nothing bigger than one finger, just at the entrance to the vagina. And this is a classic situation where lots of lubrication will make everything feel better. Don't be afraid of making a mess.

The Astounding Vagina

Vaginas may be short, narrow, tight, long, spacious, wide, soft, big, sensitive, hard, round, muscular, or any combination of these. They can expand and contract very considerably in size. It is amazing how much a vagina may change its texture and shape in a short space of time, depending on the mood of its owner or how it's being stimulated. I strongly recommend that you investigate this phenomenon on yourself, using your own fingers to feel inside yourself at different stages of turn-on. And I certainly recommend anyone who makes love to women to investigate this in their lovers! Hands are the most versatile and wonderful tools of lovemaking. Some women seem to balloon with fingers inside them, while other women tighten down. Some women get hard and muscular inside and other women get soft, like whipped cream. Some women fluctuate from one to the other.

The cervix (the lower part of the uterus) lies at the back of the vagina, sometimes lower or higher or to one side along the back wall. Although some women like cervical stimulation, it must be gently done. Men should always practice holding back their desire to ram it home, until the woman makes it clear that she is ready. Premature intercourse, resulting in the penis hitting the cervix, can be very painful. When a woman is aroused and her body is ready for intercourse, the back of the vagina becomes round (called "tenting"), the uterus pulls upwards, and the cervix retracts. In this position, it is out of the way. Women who are raped often suffer damage to the ligaments that hold up the cervix. This is because, due to their lack of arousal during the assault, the cervix isn't pulled out of the way, and it gets battered by the penis. This may result in prolapse of the uterus, which means that the muscles that normally hold the uterus up are unable to do so and the uterus drops down into the vagina.

Taking It Slowly

Hard, fast, deep penetration can be very hot, and there are certainly times when that is what is wanted. But not many women can take a lot of banging on the back wall of their vaginas, and they may prefer slower, more sensual penetration, at least initially. Almost all women want it slower some of the time, and there is a great deal to be said for allowing the sexual sensations to flood all the way through the body. I stress this, not because I think it is *better* than fast, hard sex, but because it is something that few people practice. Fast, hard sex is exactly that — it carries you fast and hard, so you don't really have time to let the experience sink fully into your awareness. Since so many of us are uncomfortable with explicitly sexual feelings, we may prefer to keep it that way. It wasn't until I realized how fulfilling it was to be fully open to the depth of my sexual feelings, and the connection with my partner that inevitably followed, that I was able to do sex slowly, and to revel in the exquisite delight of feeling every sensation throughout my whole body.

Deborah Sundahl describes slow, gentle genital massage that is nurturing as well as erotic:

There is a way we can learn to drop into ourselves: it requires complete physical, emotional, and mental relaxation. With a slow, gentle touch and deep breathing, we can let go and surrender into the sensations, and reach a state of arousal that is like a meditation. In that stillness, we become alive.

The G Spot

The most sensitive area of the vagina is usually the G spot. This area can be felt through the front wall of the vagina about an inch in, just behind the urethral opening. Some women report no sensation at all in the vagina. Others report different sensations of varying intensity in different areas of the vagina, and this is where fingers are the perfect instrument for searching out those wonderfully sensitive places. Try hooking your fingers under the cervix, circling the cervix, hooking your fingers behind the G spot, stroking the surface of the G spot, stroking the vaginal walls in a circle with vary-ing pressure, and moving in and out.

Some women never locate anything that corresponds to a G spot, so don't get hung up on finding it. It is much less dis-tinct in some women than in others. You are looking for a particularly erogenous area within your vagina, not some magical spot. It is a mistake to think of the G spot as an iso-lated lump, separate from the rest of your vagina or your cli-toris. It is one of several areas of erectile tissue that make up the genitals, a sensitive part of the whole female sexual anatomy, which is united by nerve endings that connect directly to the brain as well as other parts of the body.

Of the women who do recognize a G spot, some say it is bean-sized, whereas others say it is more like the size of the ball of their thumb.

It's rough and bumpy. The skin on it is like a strawberry, with pits and bumps.

My G spot feels like gills. It feels a little bit different from the rest of my vagina — it has ridges. It's bigger than an almond, more like a Brazil nut.

My G spot is about two knuckles long and one knuckle wide, and it feels like a rough sponge covered with little pockets.

I've never really tried to find it, but it isn't an immediately apparent feature of my body, and even after some years of sex-ual activity it appears I haven't found it.

I have no experience of a so-called G spot and no interest in it either.

Location, Location, Location

You should be able to feel your G spot clearly if you just rub your fingers across that area. Because it is erectile tissue, it will begin to swell. Mine quickly develops hard ridges at the lower end (the end closer to the entrance of my vagina) when I rub it. However, it isn't clearly defined: I couldn't say where it ends or begins.

Direct stimulation of the G spot can be so intense that some women experience it as pain, so please proceed gently! Other women will have trouble differentiating it from any other part of the vagina. But stroking the G spot may cause an orgasm very quickly, and it causes some women to ejaculate. I discuss female ejaculation in detail in the next chapter.

Because an erect penis doesn't bend (much), it doesn't stimulate the G spot as well as fingers. (I'm happy to report that all but one of the men who responded to the questionnaire say they regularly used their fingers for penetration.) If you do want a penis or a dildo to stimulate the G spot, it is a little more effective in certain positions, in particular when the woman is on all fours or bending over, facing away from her partner. Different positions can make a tremendous difference to a woman's enjoyment, so I recommend that you experiment. The best method I have found for locating the G spot is to lie on your back, have someone insert two fingers into your vagina and curl them up towards the belly, as though using a beckoning motion. This catches the back of the G spot. From there the fingers should be pulled forward out of the vagina. That way you know you have had your G spot stroked by the tips of the fingers.

*That feeling of fingers rubbing along my G spot is just fantas-
tic, and after I first experienced it (which was, of course, with
women), that really added a powerful dimension to orgasm that
hadn't been there before. A penis just doesn't do it.*

*The first time I really became aware of my G spot was when I
started having sex with women. I mean, I must have been having my G spot stimulated with men but I never knew it. Becoming aware of G spot stimulation and doing anal stimulation are
what made me have vaginal orgasms.*

*How does it feel when someone touches my G spot? I think I'm
gonna die. It's hot but it isn't a temperature — it's a pressure;
it's not nice and sweet; it's not like kissing. It sorta has fangs.
It's really visceral and intense.*

*There is a kind of unlocalized general, pleasant sensation, but
it's hard to pin down "there's the spot."*

Toys

There are many things with which to penetrate a vagina, but
please use common sense. Some vegetables work well. Do
not use a plastic bottle without a lid because there is a possibility that you may create suction and then you'll be unable to
get the bottle out. Do not use anything with sharp edges, or
anything made of glass, which might break. Do not use
anything round like a ball that might be difficult to retrieve. If
you want to experiment, go to a good sex store, or get a high-
quality sex catalog, and buy something specifically made for
the purpose. There is an enormous variety of dildoes: short,
small, fat, wide, thin, long, S-shaped, to mention a few. They
come in many different sizes and shapes and colors. Some

are curved at the end to get at the G spot more easily. Some are designed to look like a real penis and scrotum, but they can be made to represent all kinds of things, from dolphins to corn on the cob, from a fist to a woman's body. They are generally made from rubber, silicone, or plastic-related substances, but they can also be made from metal or wood. I have a friend who made several from driftwood. Obviously, plastic and silicone are the safest because they are perfectly smooth and easily cleaned. If you use anything made of wood or any other substance, please make sure it won't leave splinters or cause scraping or tearing! It must feel completely smooth to your hand, or better still, your tongue. To ensure cleanliness, which is vital if you plan to use more than one orifice, or have more than one partner, it is best to use a condom on *anything* used for penetration. Believe me, it is far easier to remove and replace a condom than it is to go into the bathroom and wash the object in question.

I find putting on a condom very erotic. I love watching fingers unrolling it.

A dildo can be wielded by hand, or, if it has a suitable flange, it can be "strapped on," using an apparatus to attach it somewhere on the body . Usually this is for attaching it in the groin area, but harnesses are being made so that the dildo can be attached to your leg, or your belly, or even your forehead. While this may seem bizarre, it gives rise to some interesting possibilities.

A harness that straps a dildo onto your groin usually consists of a couple of straps that go around each buttock, a strap round the waist, and a piece at the front where you slide the dildo through. It is held by a metal or rubber ring. (So you have to have a ring of the right size for the diameter of your dildo). Note that you cannot strap on a dildo unless it has a flange to prevent it sliding all the way through the ring.

To Use a Dildo . . . or Not Use a Dildo

Let me philosophize before I go any further. The average reader is probably convulsing with laughter, secretly or openly, at the idea of strapping on a dildo. The average old-fashioned lesbian (in the event that she reads this book), knowing that hands and mouths are by far the most versatile instruments for giving a woman pleasure, is shaking her head in hopeless amazement, and saying, "Why would anyone want to try to copy such a useless piece of equipment as a *penis?*" And the average heterosexual (who ought to be reading this book) is saying, "My god, what is she talking about, surely only lesbians need to use *dildoes?*" Neither of them can imagine keeping a straight face long enough to actually get the thing on, much less use it.

I can't imagine anything more ridiculous than a woman wearing a dildo.

I used to be one of the lesbians who couldn't understand why anyone would want to try to copy a penis. What changed my mind? I finally allowed myself to admit that penises fascinate me — not just the physical penis itself (which fascinates me in the same way a vagina does: it's an extraordinary body part, with a mind of its own), but the power that is associated with having a penis. I started playing with dildoes as hand-held objects because I had a lover who liked the sensation of something long and hard inside her, and she asked me to use one. There did seem to be times when a dildo could do things a hand could not. The same lover finally persuaded me to strap on. I struggled with my feelings around the absurdity of it all; I finally accepted that she really wanted it and I really wanted to please her, so I obliged. Still, it was another three years before I could see someone with a dildo strapped on without having to suppress the desire to laugh. They do look ridiculous (but then I used to think that about real penises back in the days when I played around with them).

Now that I take dildoes seriously, I have lots of fun with them. There is still, and always will be, a huge place in my life and my cunt for hands. However, strapping on has added a new dimension to my love life. One of the great advantages of strapping on a dildo is that it leaves your hands free to do other things. But much more than that physical factor is the psychological factor: there is just something quite different and very enjoyable about having an appendage attached to my groin. It is extremely suggestive. It need not be a blatant visual, although the visuals with a dildo can be wonderful. It can be a bulge tucked inside a pair of jeans, or even under a skirt if you want to get really kinky, or a hard phallus pressing against your belly. You can even buy dildoes that ejaculate. The gender-bending aspect of a woman with a penis is

intriguing, and the particular pelvic motions that come naturally when you are wearing a dildo are also interesting. All in
all, it is an experience worth trying if you can keep a straight
(pun intended) face.

Ode to the Dildo

Although hands are certainly more dexterous than penises,
if what you want is to be penetrated with something long,
then hands might not do it for you. Dildoes are quite versatile: for instance, they can be heated. Place a dildo in a pan
of just-boiled water before using it. Nothing relaxes and
delights the muscles of the vagina as fast as a hot dildo. It is
an experience every woman should have at least once in
her lifetime.

Among the numerous advantages of dildoes is that they
are always there, and always hard, when you want them.
They never get tired, they never get soft, they never get diseases (although they can carry them and you must make
sure you wash them thoroughly, or use condoms, or both).
They are never in the way: when you tire of them you can
happily fling them across the room. (Be careful they don't fly
out of an open window by accident, or passersby might be
startled by a flying dildo.) Buy several of different shapes and
sizes, and have a selection lined up for the evening. You can
purchase blow-up dildoes attached to a hand-held bulb to
enlarge them once they're in place. You never need to worry
about your lover's penis being too small or too big or too soft
or too unreliable again. And by the way, you can get dildoes

that your boyfriend or husband can slide over his own penis, either because he has trouble getting an erection or because you want something bigger. Oh, the wonders of modern technology!

If I were a man I think I might be alarmed at the idea that such an important part of my body could be so easily replaced with a lump of plastic. Let me reassure you, there are things a dildo cannot do. They haven't yet invented one that smells or tastes like a man, or one that can reproduce the experience of a penis going from soft to hard.

You may be wondering how the wearer of the dildo can enjoy it, for surely they have no sensation. How do they know they are in the right place at the right time? Skillful use of a strapped-on dildo requires a bit of practice, probably about as much as skillful use of a penis. You may be surprised at how quickly you become accustomed to the feel of a dildo that is in the right place. And there are all kinds of things you can do to make sure it turns you on, such as positioning it so that the base of it stimulates your clitoris, or wearing a small vibrator or another dildo inside you, so that you get plenty of stimulation as you move. The thrusting motion and the feel of the dildo against the pelvis is enough for many women. I know a number of women who come while they are wearing a strap-on: by jerking off using their own hand or someone else's; by penetrating someone; or by having someone suck them off. Some women expect to come this way, and it is their favorite form of sex. Whether it is from the physical stimulation or the psychological effects, who knows? And who cares?

Coming when I'm strapped on is somewhat tenuous. Getting there is completely dependent on her reactions, her movements, sounds, arousal, need, desire. But if I become too focused on her having an orgasm, the potential I feel building in me to have one will fall by the wayside. If I keep that balance, soon the feeling of potential becomes a feeling of certainty and then automatic thrusting takes over and I usually roar and bellow as I come. This kind of orgasm seems to go on much longer than the ones I have from masturbating or from being made love to.

I should make it clear that just because a woman experiments with strap-on dildoes does not mean she wants to be a man. Most women have no desire to have a permanent penis. What they are doing is playing with the fantasy.

Other Orifices

Of course the vagina is not the only place on the body that can be penetrated pleasurably. There are other body cavities that are used for sexual pleasure, such as the mouth and the anus. Anal penetration is discussed in following chapter.

The mouth is also an erogenous zone. There are lots of things you can have done to your mouth, or can do to your partner's mouth: simply stroking lips with a wet finger, or a finger with wet lips can be intensely arousing. But you can go a lot further than that: you can use your mouth all over someone's body and you can use various parts of your body, including temporary parts of your body like dildoes, in or on someone's mouth. Many people find it uncomfortable to have something large in their mouths, but it does not have to be large, and, to be erotic, **it should never be forced down the throat**.

Jesse recently came from having her fingers in her lover's mouth:

We'd been playing around for a while and we were both very aroused. She was licking and sucking my fingers. I told her not to move, and I slowly slid my fingers deep into her mouth until I felt the incredible softness at the back of her throat spasm around my fingertips. I held still, totally absorbed in the amazing thing happening between us, and my orgasm just surfaced from deep within me, bursting out in a roar.

The possible variations of sexual play are endless. We forget them when we focus on what we think we're meant to be doing, when we get stuck on a limited concept of what sex is, and when we fear other people's judgments. I hope this chapter will open your mind to new ways of perceiving sex as a delightfully limitless form of play.

12

CHAPTER

Ejaculation, Fisting, and Anal Sex

I don't know what causes me to ejaculate. It's happened very rarely — only as part of a long, intense bout of lovemaking (usually in the first few months of a relationship). I find it slightly embarrassing, though as I get very wet anyway I'm not sure it's that noticeable to anyone else.

What follows are discussions of some of the lesser-known possibilities in sexual play, not because I think everyone ought to be doing them, but because information on them is so limited. And these activities can be enormously pleasurable.

The G Spot and Ejaculation

The existence of the urethral sponge, or G spot, and the female ejaculation that is associated with it, are still barely acknowledged and only reluctantly accepted by many people, including many physicians. Why not? Surely a phenomenon as obvious as ejaculation would be noticed? Not by a society that has ignored and denigrated women and their sexuality for centuries. Female ejaculation was mentioned by Aristotle, so it was known in ancient times, and it is commonly acknowledged in some present day cultures. The South Pacific Trobriand Islanders described female ejaculation to Western anthropologists who, because of their ignorance, assumed that they were speaking of urination (*The G Spot*). The Batoro people, of Uganda, don't consider a woman eligible for marriage until she can spray the wall, and the older women of the tribe teach her how to do so (*The G Spot*). The implications of this are significant: obviously women can ejaculate with some force. Would we all ejaculate if it were expected of us?

Ejaculation may be more common among lesbians.

During twenty years of straight sex I never once experienced ejaculation with a man; now, with women, I ejaculate nearly 100 percent of the time.

This could be because she is more orgasmic with women, or that the kind of sex she does with women is more conducive to ejaculation, or both. It is also possible for a woman to be unaware she is ejaculating.

After we'd been having sex, there was always a big wet spot in the bed, and I always thought it was him. Much later, another man told me that he could feel me squeezing fluid past his penis when we were having intercourse, and I realized that the wet spot was me.

One woman responded to the questionnaire with: No, she didn't ejaculate. Then she crossed out her "No" and wrote:

Well, this is interesting! I was completely unaware of ejaculating until I filled in your questionnaire. Then I talked with my partner, who informed me, with surprise, that I didn't realize that I ejaculate profusely when highly orgasmic, usually with oral stimulation. I said, "I thought all that wetness was just spit!" "No, no, no!" said he.

What Is It and Where Does It Come From?

When we do notice it, we may think we are urinating, and if our lovers don't know any better, they may well support us in this assumption. While there are a few women who lose bladder control during sexual activity, female ejaculation is *not* incontinence. The chemical composition of the fluid that is released is different from urine, although it does contain varying (usually small) quantities of the same substances as urine. It is similar in composition to male ejaculatory fluid, without the semen. It appears to be produced by the paraurethral glands (or Skene's glands), which lie within the erectile tissue of the urethral sponge. The ducts of these glands empty into the urethral canal. Because the male prostate gland is homologous to the urethral sponge, the G spot is sometimes referred to as the G spot prostate.

However, because it has not been documented at all until recently, many doctors have no idea that female ejaculation is a perfectly normal sexual response, and not an aberration. Women who tend to ejaculate profusely may prevent themselves from doing so, thus censoring their sexuality in order to avoid dealing with negative reactions. Female ejaculation has often been misdiagnosed as urinary stress incontinence. The solution offered for this problem was often surgery. (There is little incentive for a woman to question a doctor's diagnosis when she is not only embarrassed by the condition, but is also desperate to be normal.) There is no way to know how many women have had unnecessary operations, because there is no way of discerning, in retrospect, whether these patients were ejaculating or, in fact, peeing. It is time for female ejaculation to be recognized for what it is: a completely normal sexual response.

Female ejaculatory fluid is thin and usually clear, although sometimes it has a yellow tinge; it may also be whitish. It does not leave a stain when it dries. One woman, who went to the trouble of collecting hers, says:

My ejaculate contains a visible suspension that, over time, will precipitate. This precipitate appears to be whitish and somewhat mucosal, consistent with the type of secretion produced by the male prostate gland.

The ejaculate appears to be expelled from the urethral opening (as is male ejaculate). Women report that it has different odors, varying from sweet and sexy to a little fishy, but they all say it is odorless when it dries. You may realize you are ejaculating if you find you are not quite so well lubed down there, even though you are still very excited. The ejaculate is watery and has the same effect as water: things don't slide on it, and it tends to wash away the lubrication. It is quite unlike the thick, clear, or whitish slippery secretion that is produced in fairly small quantities by an excited vagina.

The fact is, we still know very little about female ejaculation, and about the range of possible sexual responses. The first time I experienced a woman ejaculating, I thought it was the hottest thing that had happened to me in a long time, and I didn't care whether it was pee or not. She hit me in the chest with a powerful spray of fluid as I knelt between her legs with my fingers inside her. I was astounded. This particular lover would regularly soak the bed with her ejaculations. Sometimes she would flood, and sometimes she would squirt. I usually left the sheets drawn back after we'd made love, so that the bed would dry. The fluid never left a stain or an odor once it was dry. One day we were coming out of the bedroom when a couple of friends of mine were in the passageway. I saw one of them look at the bed and then clutch her lover's arm in excitement. "Look, Jane, someone else does it! I'm not the only one!" She knew exactly where that wet spot came from. Like many women, she was embarrassed about her tendency to ejaculate, and very happy to find out that she was indeed not the only one.

This is how one man feels about it:

I love to help a woman explore her capacity to ejaculate, and I love to make it happen, and I love to be covered in it when it does.

Who? When? How Much?

Some women apparently never ejaculate at all; some have always ejaculated since they first became actively sexual; some ejaculate only with a lot of penetration; some women teach themselves to do it; others try to learn without success; some women squirt fluid; others just flood.

What is responsible for the variation? One hypothesis suggests that it may depend on the number of paraurethral glands in the urethral sponge: some women may have thirty or more, while others may have only five or six. One of the men I spoke with claims that there is a correlation between the size of the G spot and ejaculation. According to his theory, the larger and more well-defined a woman's G spot is (which may well relate to the number of glands and ducts in the urethral sponge), the more likely she is to ejaculate.

The strength of the PC muscle may also play a part, although I know women with very strong pelvic muscles who don't ejaculate.

The more fit and muscular I am, due to weight training and lots of pelvic tilt exercises, the easier and more intense are my ejaculatory orgasms.

The stimulus that causes ejaculation to occur varies from woman to woman, as do all sexual responses, and it also varies according to her psychological and emotional state. A number of women report that the same kind of stimulation will sometimes fail to make them ejaculate at all, and at other times make them flood the bed. A few women can consciously make it happen, but most can't. Several women have commented that they associate ejaculation with being relaxed, and I believe this is a key factor. In this sense it's a different experience from a purely clitoral orgasm, which often seems to require some preliminary tension.

With a G spot orgasm I find there is a need to relax that isn't necessary for a clitoral orgasm. I have to remember to relax, to let the sensation go up inside.

It is also possible that ejaculation occurs in some women

and not in others due to a range of anatomical differences. Anatomical variations in the genital region are not unusual, and it seems reasonable to suppose that there is a gradation of ability to ejaculate, related to small differences in the equipment a person is born with.

I ejaculate frequently just because I am aroused, without any physical stimulation of my G spot.

Oral sex is a fairly common method of incitement. So are vibrators. Joy taught herself to ejaculate by experimenting at home until she found the right combination of stimuli to do it herself. She uses a strong vibrator, but finds the combination of deep penetration and vibrator is more reliable. Linda uses a heavy-duty vibrator pressed against her vulva, angled slightly upwards.

But in the majority of cases, ejaculation seems to result from intense sexual arousal involving direct G spot stimulation. Laura can ejaculate without being touched at all, but, according to her lover, she ejaculates more copiously when she is being stimulated by fingers hooked behind her G spot.

Some women only ejaculate with penetration. Quite a few of the women I spoke with were in their forties and had started to ejaculate recently. Indeed, women such as Terry, Jesse, and myself all associate the experience of ejaculation with fisting, or at least with heavy penetration. However, it may be simply that we are at an age and a place in our lives when we are more open and relaxed, mentally and physically, thus allowing us to experience new sensations.

The most typical and most gratifying ejaculatory orgasm I

know is through strapping on and having "intercourse" with a woman. When a partner is not available, I ejaculate through male-like masturbation, either by simulating intercourse (e.g., humping a pillow) or by jerking off (wearing a strap-on).

So you see, for me, and I assume I am not alone, ejaculation is more akin to the type of ejaculatory response experienced by men; there is no direct involvement of the vagina.

If your partner sits between your legs, he or she can feel your G spot by inserting two fingers and then curling the fingers up as though making a beckoning motion. For most women, that is the position that will stimulate them to ejaculate, although it may be too intense, producing a strong sensation of the desire to urinate. This need to urinate may be misleading: many women report feeling the need to pee just prior to ejaculation, when, in fact, that intense swelling feeling is the desire to ejaculate. It may be that women who would otherwise ejaculate stop themselves from doing so, because they think they are going to pee. It is possible to retrain yourself to experience urination anxiety as a pleasurable sexual response. You can do this by sitting on the toilet, emptying your bladder completely, and then stimulating your G spot until you feel the need to pee again. You will probably find you don't actually need to. Every time you think you do, let yourself do so, and then resume touching your G spot.

The amount of ejaculate varies considerably from event to event and woman to woman. Some women may consistently ejaculate, but only in small amounts. Other women ejaculate copiously. The amount of fluid that can be produced is phenomenal, and a few women can carry on for an hour or even more.

Multiple, back-to-back ejaculations do not decrease the volume of ejaculate produced: the fourth or fifth ejaculation can be just as voluminous as the first.

One of my current companions is a "hair trigger." A few licks and tickles and a bit of heavy pressure and massage with two or three fingers, and she's primed for a series of flowing orgasms that flood the bed (impervious groundcloth under the sheets leaves three to five sodden towels and actual pools that we end up rolling around in). It always amazes me the quantity of fluid that she is capable of producing and how quickly she can recover and go again.

The Relationship of Orgasm to Ejaculation

Ejaculation is sometimes simultaneous with orgasm, but definitely not for all women all of the time. Some said it was not related to orgasms. Quite a number of the women I questioned said that it commonly occurred just before orgasm, but for some it occurred afterwards. For women who have multiple orgasms, it can be quite difficult to distinguish between what is an orgasm and what is the plateau between. However, this woman is very clearly able to differentiate, and finds that ejaculation is a kind of orgasm in itself:

I have always ejaculated, although I didn't have a clitoral orgasm until I was forty-four. Nowadays I ejaculate before or after a clitoral orgasm, not during. I can tell when I am about to ejaculate. It's a buildup to a climax and then a sudden relief of tension, satisfying in itself but quite different from the deep orgasm I have with clitoral stimulation, which is like a flow of energy exploding from the sex center with waves up the spine and down to the fingers and toes, which then gradually ebbs away deliciously.

The woman quoted below is clear that ejaculation enhances her orgasms:

Ejaculatory orgasms are far, far more intense and decidedly more satisfying than any nonejaculatory orgasm I've ever had.

One woman says that she loses all interest in and desire for sex after she has ejaculated, even though she doesn't experience the ejaculation as an orgasm in itself:

I ejaculate from vaginal stimulation only, when my vagina is dilated and very wet. The ejaculation makes me too wet to orgasm and everything relaxes; sensation is gone and I hardly notice any further stimulation.

The Power of Ejaculation

Freed from the embarrassment of thinking they are incontinent, most women find ejaculation very pleasurable. Deborah Sundahl, who has produced a video called *How To Female Ejaculate*, connects its physical and emotional release with a deeply cleansing spiritual surrender.

The first time Linda ejaculated a sizeable quantity of fluid, she felt that the expulsion of the fluid was directly connected to her rage against a man who had abused her:

I started having orgasm after orgasm and I got to the ninth one, and all of a sudden I shot out an ounce or two of fluid. I had ejaculated before but only a little bit, nothing like this. While I was masturbating I'd been thinking about this man who had sexually and emotionally abused me, and I'd been cursing him and yelling at him. It was like the ejaculation was a huge emotional release. I still had more orgasms inside me, and I still felt angry. I was gnashing my teeth, so I carried on and had three or four more, and then on the fourteenth one I shot out almost exactly the same quantity of fluid as the first time. I was so amazed — here I found I could shoot out all that fluid, I mean where did it come from?

My personal experience is that I never know when I have done it, and other women say the same thing: there were times when they had what they thought was the sensation of ejaculation, but there didn't appear to be any ejaculate; and there were other times when they were surprised to discover that they had soaked the bed.

It's not always simultaneous with an orgasm, and sometimes it feels like a whole other kind of orgasm. Other times I don't know I'm doing it until I find there's a big puddle. I squirt, I don't flood; I once shot a couple of feet at least. Sometimes both me and my lover think I'd be ejaculating but I'm not.

Even women who had been doing it all their lives said that sometimes they only knew they were ejaculating because there were certain kinds of stimulation that always made it happen.

Victoria and Judy, who both ejaculate on a regular basis, commonly push out whatever is inside them — fingers, dildo, penis, fist — by contracting their vaginal muscles very hard when they ejaculate. If they're not able to do that, then they can't squirt (though they may flood and seep) because the fluid cannot escape; and perhaps also because they cannot contract the vaginal walls.

Vaginal Fisting

Fisting is an activity that involves one person inserting his or her whole hand into another person's anus or vagina. It is as intense an experience as it sounds. **Please — do not attempt it until you have spoken with someone who has done it, and read about how to do it! Serious, permanent injury is a possible consequence of fisting inexpertly done!**

Vaginal fisting is a common practice among some lesbians. It is presumably less common amongst heterosexuals because they are less likely to use their hands in sexual play. Men also tend to have larger fists. In theory, anyone can fist anyone else, no matter what their sexual orientation. It is not an activity that is limited to women who have had babies, have large vaginas, and have lovers with small hands, although all these may be advantages. The only essential prerequisite is the desire coupled with the belief that it is not only possible but enjoyable. Many of us have a psychological block against fisting because we think it will be painful. In fact, when our bodies are ready for it, there is no pain associated with fisting, only pleasure.

Nevertheless, as a concept, fisting is totally out of the question to many of us — and there was certainly a time when it was unimaginable to me. I could not visualize comfortably accommodating more than two or, at most, three fingers in my vagina. There are still times when this is true for me. The first time I conceived the possibility that I might take someone's whole hand inside me, I dismissed it at once. At that time, my lover had had a baby, but I had not. So, I reasoned, my vagina was not likely to be able to expand enough to take a fist. But . . . lo and behold, a few months went by, and we got close to it several times, until I got frightened and tightened up. She kept telling me I was huge inside. I knew what *she* was capable of: her vagina opened up into a huge, moist cave. Was mine doing the same thing? One day when we had been making love for a while, I put my fingers inside my own vagina, and sure enough, there was plenty of room in there. Pretty soon thereafter she slipped her whole hand inside me. There was a moment of cramping and then a blissfully intense sensation. I had never felt so delightfully filled up.

The vagina is designed to expand to allow a baby's head and body to pass through it, and most newborns' heads are bigger than most adult's fists, and some women's fists are smaller than some men's penises. Men should remember that they tend to have big fists, and **nothing should *ever* be forced into the vagina.**

What makes vaginal fisting possible is the ability of the vagina to change its shape when it is stimulated in the right kinds of ways. It is normal for a vagina to "balloon," that is, the muscles of the vaginal walls contract very tightly and pull away from each other, forming a spacious, round, hard-walled cave. In the previous chapter, I mentioned "tenting," which is apparently the early stages of ballooning. A ballooned vagina is an ideal receptacle for something round like a fist.

I personally find that my vagina alternates quite rapidly between this ballooned state and the opposite state, where the walls turn completely soft, like whipped cream, and the whole vagina closes in on itself. The walls are so soft at that point that it's almost as though the vagina is trying to suck something in. It's like putting your hand inside a jellyfish that doesn't sting!

Someone who is not already perfectly comfortable with deep penetration (five fingers) is not going to be able to take a fist, so don't even try. But if you have been enjoying deep penetration and can take all five of your partner's fingers without discomfort, then slipping past the third set of knuckles is quite possible. However, you do need to be in an emotional space where you can completely relax. You must trust your partner. Make sure she or he fully understands how to do it. Being fisted requires a profound level of surrender. Set aside time for foreplay that really turns you on. Give your partner plenty of verbal feedback about how it feels and what you want. Be prepared for a little cramping the first time you are fisted. **Stop at once if you experience any severe pain.** The same warnings apply to fisting as to all sexual activities: be willing to let go of the idea if it becomes uncomfortable or painful. It does no good for your head to decide today will be the day if your body is not in agreement. Put aside your agenda, and don't be in a hurry. You can always try again another day.

There have been times when my head wants my vagina to take a fist, and my body has refused it. Why my body sometimes refuses a fist is a matter for conjecture since my body doesn't form words except under instruction from my head. But I would say it is because there are some unresolved emotional issues with my lover; usually issues that have nothing to do with sex, and often issues that I think I have already dealt with. But my body responds on a physical level, as bodies tend to do, by not letting her in physically.

The How-to's of Vaginal Fisting

You have to be careful with fisting; there is a thin edge between what you want and what your body can take. You get so into it that you want to have a sense of something driving up through your eyeballs. You really have to trust someone to let yourself experience that. With fisting you have to consciously consent to the whole sexual experience, not just to orgasm.

If you are going to fist someone, make sure your fingernails are short and smooth, and you have no hangnails. Remove rings, bracelets, and wristwatches. The contact between your hand and your partner's vaginal walls will be much greater than when you're just using a couple of fingers, so a latex glove (or other kind) is necessary for safer sex, and may in any case ensure that you don't abrade your lover. If you insist on having long nails, put cotton balls in the fingertips of the glove before you put it on. Use lots of lube, approximately three times as much as you think you need. Apply it to the fist, though it's a good idea to smear some around the vagina as well. **Don't hesitate to stop and apply more any time you think you may need it.**

The entrance to the vagina must be relaxed, since that is normally the tightest part. There are two rings of muscle that control the entrance to the vagina, and the inner ring is the part that tenses up.

Take your time. Make yourselves comfortable. You could have your partner lie on her back with her legs over the end of the bed while you sit on a chair between her legs. If you arrange yourself so that you are sitting a little lower than the fistee, you won't have to bend your wrist so much, and the angle of penetration is slightly up towards her belly rather than down towards her spine, which she may find more comfortable. The fistee could also be on all fours, facing away from the fister.

Spend as much time as you need — hours, if necessary — just playing around, with three or four or all five fingers up to the second set of knuckles. If you're smart, you will not be attempting this unless you are accustomed to this kind of play already. At this stage, keep your fingers together and straight, or only slightly bent. Keep your thumb curled in so that it lies in the center of your palm. If the fistee is not happy with five fingers, then don't press on!

Follow your partner's direction as to when to push and when not to push. Be sensitive to her body language. Tune in to her responses and watch her facial expressions.

When, finally, your third set of knuckles slides in past the tight point, let your hand close into a fist, preferably with your thumb tucked inside. At this juncture your partner will want you to hold still inside since she may experience a little cramping. Usually this will pass within a few seconds; if it doesn't, remove your fist and try again another day. You can try some clitoral stimulation, as this sometimes eases the cramping, but if you are both beginners, it is wiser to withdraw.

Invite feedback, and allow your partner to direct the action. Clitoral stimulation at any point during the process may feel very good. Lightly stroking or fluttering your hand on the belly just above the pubic bone can also be very pleasing; so can stroking her thighs, buttocks, and nipples.

It's a completion of experience, having my hand in another woman's vagina.

Removing your fist when you're finished is often easier said than done, especially as your partner may tighten down if she orgasms. And after she comes once or twice or more, your hand may begin to feel as if it's being sliced off at the wrist. You can either time the removal of your hand with the final contractions of an orgasm, at which point she is usually pushing out, or you can wait until she's finished and starts to relax, and then ease your hand out as best you can.

I recall one time when I was being fisted and the fist got stuck, and it wasn't until we started joking about having to spend the rest of our lives that way, and laughing hilariously, that we were able to come unstuck.

What do you do with your fist while it's in there? That depends very much on your partner and the size of your fist. If you have a large fist or she has a small vagina, you may not be able to move much, and she may simply get off on the sensation of being filled up; she may not want you to move at all, and your attempts to move may cause cramping. But if you have a small fist or she has a large vagina, you may be able to move quite a bit. Moving sideways, to and fro, or round and round, even very slightly, can be very exciting. Be careful not to push hard into the vagina since you may hit her cervix. If you have lots of room, try extending your fingers and stroking the walls of her vagina in various places with your knuckles and fingertips. You can also try just expanding and tightening your fist.

If your partner is on all fours, facing away from you, the sensations of movement inside are quite different. Some people definitely prefer being fisted in this position.

Vaginal Fisting and Orgasms

Being fisted is certainly an incredible experience, and the orgasms that result are often very intense. Along with the extraordinary feelings of trust and openness, several women I spoke with experience a sense of helplessness and immobility, which they enjoy. For others, it is not vulnerability but aggression that comes to the surface.

When I am being fisted I feel very aggressive, very primal, very "animalistic." I get incredibly loud and I growl. It is probably the only time I am 100 percent selfish in sex and I think if anyone tried to step in and stop it, I would snarl and snap like a wolf whose kill is being threatened! Also, my orgasms are different: less of a spike upward to orgasm and more of a long, slow ramp, indescribably intense and pleasurable with a hint of pain. — Mary

When I am the fister, it makes me feel incredibly powerful! I feel like I am inside her soul, like there is total spiritual communion with her; to experience her complete surrender to me;

to smell, hear, and see her arousal; to feel her opening to my hand, to my will! — Mary

It arouses a feeling so intense in me that I feel as if I'm going to explode from the inside . . . and the orgasm I have is not the same as a clitoral orgasm, it's much more intensified . . . it feels like I can't take any more, but I don't want the feeling to stop. — Denice

The experience of fisting is the purest transfer of kundalini, and the most intense intimacy, that I know. — Catherine A. Liszt

For a while now, I've recognized that I finally "learned" how to meditate during my quest to be fisted. That sense of relaxation, of concentration and not-concentration, of openness, of whole-ness. . . I was somewhat floored when I first realized that what I was doing was, essentially, meditating, and that this was why the sensation was so much more intense and fulfilling.

I really couldn't figure out why fisting was so different from other types of penetration, why that particular type of openness was something I was so intensely drawn to, until I thought about kundalini. The openness is the same as I get during my medita-tion/masturbation exercises, but there's something further . . . the degree of connection . . . yes, it is like being touched, inside, not in my body but in my energy stream. It's touch that goes beyond the physical into a different kind of sensation. — Renee

This is by no means a complete introduction to fisting. If fisting is an activity that interests you, I suggest reading *A Hand in the Bush: The Fine Art of Vaginal Fisting*, by Deborah Addington, published by Greenery Press.

Anal Sex

Many women find the idea of anal sex off-putting, and usually it is because we are concerned about hygiene, or because it seems so invasive, or because we expect it to be painful. Transmission of AIDS and other diseases such as hepatitis can certainly occur through anal sex more quickly than through other forms of sexual play, but latex or nitrile gloves and condoms are effective barriers.

Anal sex should not hurt, and if it does, stop! The anus is a taboo area of the body, and we may simply not wish to deal with the feelings that come up when someone touches us there. On the other hand, it is exactly that taboo quality that attracts others to it.

The anus is full of nerve endings, which can make for very pleasurable sensations. If you wish to try anal sex, the same rules apply as for vaginal fisting: relax, take it slowly, use plenty of lube, give and be willing to receive feedback. **(Using plenty of lubrication for anal sex is not an option, it is essential**, since the anus does not provide any natural lubrication.) To begin with, you may simply want to spend time stroking the outside of the anus, which can be extremely erotic in itself, without any penetration at all.

The art in anal penetration is learning to relax the anal sphincter, and most people find this does need practice and trust, so don't expect to be able to perform anal penetration with more than one finger in one day. It may take months to be ready and willing to accept something as large as a penis (even a fairly small one). There is no hurry. The best preparation is doing it a little at a time, both alone and with a partner.

Oral stimulation of the anus is another option. However, **ingestion of fecal matter can cause life-threatening**

diseases, so always use a protective barrier before you proceed. Use scissors to cut a glove open on one side so that your tongue will fit in the thumbhole; apply some lube to the skin, to increase sensitivity. You may also use plastic wrap.

Due to the ease of transmitting disease during anal play, I strongly recommend using a glove for anal penetration with a finger or fingers. It is a matter of basic hygiene: if you encounter fecal matter in there (which is fairly common, and certainly isn't the end of the world), you can simply rip the glove off when you're done, turning it inside out as you do so. Using a glove can also ensure that you don't accidentally use an unwashed hand in the vagina. Introducing even minute amounts of fecal matter into the vagina will almost certainly lead to a vaginal, bladder, or kidney infection.

Gloves also protect you from any other disease contamination that might occur; the lining of the rectum is very thin, and minute tears can occur quite easily. Be careful that you don't insert anything remotely sharp-edged into the anus, and that includes your fingernails. Make absolutely sure that your nails are short and smooth.

Of course, you can use other objects for anal penetration: butt plugs especially for that purpose can be acquired from any sex store. They are usually made of plastic or silicone, in a variety of shapes and sizes. Even if you use a condom on them, they should be thoroughly washed after use, with an antibacterial soap. Obviously you can use a dildo or a penis. Another major warning is in order here: **never use anything breakable or sharp, and never use anything that does not have a flange to prevent it going all the way up**

inside the rectum, where you won't be able to retrieve it.
If you get something stuck up inside, you will have to go
to the emergency room to have it removed. And that won't
be fun.

Once you have inserted something inside the anus, you
may want to hold it still, especially if you are a beginner.
Sometimes the sensation of moving in and out can make the
receiver want to empty his or her bowels. The anal sphincter
responds automatically by tightening up, and this can
become uncomfortable.

Anal fisting (called handballing in some gay male circles)
is not something I have ever done, but I know a few women,
and a number of men, who do it and love it. I reckon anyone
who allows themselves to be anally fisted has perfected the
art of relaxation.

Whether you are engaging in anal sex or vaginal penetration, you want to try to make sure your bowels are at least
fairly empty, in order to ensure comfort for both you and
your partner. Intense penetration squashes things around in
there, and if you're trying to prevent yourself from going
while you're trying to come, you will experience some conflict. On the other hand, you might not care what happens. It
certainly doesn't have to matter in a practical sense if you do
lose control of your bladder or your bowels. These are, after
all, perfectly normal, natural bodily functions, and anything
can be cleaned up.

But most of us would be mortified with embarrassment in
the wake of such an "accident" while we are making love. So
visit the restroom before you have sex, or during if you need

to. If you're going to have anal sex, wash around your anus first, and if you feel the need, you can always do an enema to clean out your bowels. Or you can do an enema as part of your play.

The most important thing is not to do sex when you feel uncomfortable about it; your partner can wait. If you have a date and you anticipate some heavy duty kind of penetration, use common sense and don't eat a big meal just beforehand. If you know you tend to feel a little bloated in the morning, then don't have sex in the mornings. Take care of your general health: eat well, and make sure there is plenty of fiber in your diet. Do whatever you need to do to feel comfortable, and remember, we all urinate and defecate, so neither you nor your partner will die if you come into contact with a little bit of pee or poop.

Anal sex can be enormously erotic, both because the anal canal is full of sensitive nerve endings, and because it leads to a level of vulnerability that can be very rewarding.

For me, anal sex is a pathway to ecstasy. It makes sex so much more intense. The orgasms I have when I'm doing anal sex involve more of my body. They crawl up my spine.

Don't do it unless you are willing to be vulnerable, and you know that your partner will appreciate, respect, and care for you when you are in that state of vulnerability.

Some women actually prefer anal sex to vaginal sex. The G spot can be stimulated through the thin rectal wall, and the perineal sponge is stimulated directly during anal penetration; both of these are highly erogenous erectile tissue. A

very few women are able to come from anal penetration
alone, and a few more say they come more easily when they
are doing anal sex, as long as they are getting some other
kind of stimulation as well. Some women seem to find that
stimulation of the anal area relates more directly to clitoral
stimulation than vaginal stimulation does, which is not as
outlandish as it seems, when you consider that there is a
much greater concentration of nerve endings around the
anus and the clitoris than in the vagina.

*I wouldn't say I come more easily during anal sex; it is just dif-
ferent, I am more "out of control" with it.*

*Orgasms from anal sex come from a different place. I feel them
deep in my first chakra.*

*I don't know if it's the naughtiness taboo, but I find anal sex
intensely pleasurable and come a lot quicker. When I was with
men I used to prefer anal sex as it left my clitoris more accessible to my fingers. Also it didn't dull sensation, which is what
happened during vaginal penetration with men.*

This section does not pretend to be a complete guide to
anal sex. I recommend Tristan Taormino's book, *The Ultimate
Guide to Anal Sex for Women* (published by Cleis Press). This
is an excellent book for men too. Men are perfectly capable
of enjoying anal stimulation and penetration, although many
of them are also afraid of it, often more so than women are.
There are two likely reasons for this: firstly, they are afraid it
might mean they are gay. I really cannot go into how ridiculous this is, so I hope it will be enough for me to point out
that the presence of a penis is not required for anal penetration. Secondly, I think men are afraid of how vulnerable it

will make them if they admit they want anal penetration. And it will make them vulnerable, there is no doubt about that; you cannot bend over and allow someone to penetrate you and still feel that you are in control. How sad that so many men will never experience the glory of fully surrendering in total trust to another person, and so many women will never be the recipient of that trust.

13
CHAPTER

The Purpose of Orgasm

Orgasms are a great key to health and happiness. They help us to remember who we are, beyond our everyday reality. Orgasms are a path to truth and the meaning of life. — Annie Sprinkle

*M*any people have proposed many theories with regard to the social, anthropological, and biological purposes of female orgasm. These range from the obvious (that female orgasm tones the muscles that we use in childbirth) to the ridiculous. However, the unique combination of orgasm with virtually unrestricted sexual availability (we are not limited to a cycle of estrus or "heat" in order to experience sexual desire) has had, and continues to have, an overwhelming impact on our species.

In today's world, sex involves much more than our genitals and is about much more than procreation. To limit sex to making babies is as absurd and unrealistic as deciding not to use a motorized vehicle because God gave us feet to walk with. Sex can be merely functional, but it can also be an art form that gives us infinite pleasure. Who wants to live in a world that is purely functional? Beauty and joy are very important aspects of life. The variety of ways that we can express ourselves sexually is a gift, an offering from the universe. A woman can have as many different kinds of orgasms as there are ways of having sex. An orgasm can come and go in a second, or last for hours. It can be an electrical feeling on the surface of the skin, it can be a deep pounding internal sensation, it can occur in the upper body, the lower body, or throughout the whole body, and can be accompanied by an out-of-body experience. It can shake your entire being, or pass through with barely an external sign. There is no one definitive experience that we can call orgasm — there are many. Nor can we limit what arouses us sexually to a physical touch, or to a sensation in a certain part of the body.

Anyone can choose to claim her passion, and translate it into creative play, sexual or otherwise. The exceptions may be people who have been severely traumatized so that they are unable to recover positive feelings around sexual arousal; and people who suffer from severe chronic pain or illness. In general, what prevents us from embracing the full potential of our sexual desire is our fear of not being normal, and it is this, more than anything else, that we must overcome. **There is no such thing as an abnormal desire**.

What's more, there is no such thing as a normal desire! The concept of normality does not exist when it comes to what turns us on. There is no one right way of being sexual. On the contrary, there is a huge variety of sexual activities and responses, some of them stranger than your imagination could dream up, from foot fetishism to sadomasochism. A safe environment, one where the key concepts of consensu-

ality and negotiation are honored, can be created to play
with the oddest desires. What matters is that you don't
allow yourself to be swayed by the opinions of others, and
that you do not harm yourself or others. Go for what you
want: don't censor yourself or anyone else.

Inhibitions, instilled into us as we grow up, can prevent us
from getting in touch with what turns us on in the first place.
But change only needs a willingness to be open. Changes
specific to your sexuality are not so difficult to manifest as
you might think. True, you cannot make your body have an
orgasm unless it wants to. But when we give our bodies permission to change, all kinds of things become possible. This
was illustrated for me during the time it took to write this
book. I drew my close friends into my research. They
graciously accepted my calls at any time of day or night to
answer questions like: Can you feel contractions in your
vagina when you come? Do you have to stretch out your feet
when you come? How long do your orgasms normally last?
And so on.

We found that our sexual horizons have expanded simply
as a result of thinking intensely about orgasm, finding a language to express ourselves, and discovering new potentials.
We all seem to be having longer and more powerful orgasms.
Knowing what women are capable of experiencing has given
us the incentive to open up to other ways of being sexual.
Just knowing that something is possible can magically open
us to experiencing it. Discovering the range of what women
define as orgasm has encouraged us to define our own experiences differently. This new focus on familiar sensations and

experiences has made them more intense, occur more frequently, and last longer. The process of being orgasmic is constantly unfolding and evolving, if we allow it to do so. It is a journey, and the point of the process is the journey, not some mythical end product.

From Pain to Pleasure, and Beyond . . .

One of the remarkable things about the orgasmic state is how it acts as an analgesic; things we normally experience as painful may not be felt at all when we are in the throes of a climax. In *Women Who Love Sex* (Pocket Books, 1994), Gina Ogden illustrates how, during orgasm, a woman registers no pain response to a stimulus (steady pressure applied to the fingertip by an Analgesia Meter) that she was unable to tolerate only minutes beforehand. Yet her ability to experience a sensual touch (a hair-thin filament brushed across the back of her hand) is increased.

Gina Ogden, Beverley Whipple, and other renowned sex researchers have done a number of controlled studies that prove the remarkable power of orgasm to raise a woman's pain threshold (*Annual Review of Sex Research*, Volume VI, 1995, Komisaruk and Whipple). Apparently, the greater the pleasure, the stronger the analgesic effect.

In *Extended Sexual Orgasm*, the authors describe a group of arthritics who experience some freedom from pain for half an hour following orgasm. The question is, would they be free from pain for longer periods if they had extended orgasms? The Brauers claim that in some cases all of the following problems have been alleviated, if not cured by the regular practice of ESO: headaches, neck, back, and pelvic pain, menstrual pain, arthritic pain, stomach and intestinal complaints, prostatitis, high blood pressure, asthma and bronchitis, skin eruptions, depression, fatigue, anxiety, alcoholism, insomnia, and anger.

Is it too outrageous to imagine that doctors could be prescribing orgasms instead of, or in conjunction with, pain medications? And are we capable of expanding our concept of orgasm, with its attendant benefits?

Sensual and sexual intimacy, the experience of sharing one's body with another, skin-to-skin contact, the arousal and release of orgasm — all of these can suffuse the body with pleasure and with a sense of joy, delight, love, peace, and relaxation that results in freedom from pain and tension — a different human condition. Orgasm is a building and release of tension that enervates and cleanses a person's energy, clears out blocks, and leaves the body suffused with well-being. Encouraged to allow ourselves to share our bodies, take pride in our physical selves, and integrate our experience of love on mental, emotional, and spiritual levels, through the medium of the physical body, we can live creative and joyful lives.

It seems obvious to me that the purpose of sex, and therefore orgasm, is to provide us with an opportunity to experience ecstasy; an opportunity to choose pleasure. On one level, this is about experiencing joy in life, having a good time, allowing and encouraging us to feel good. People who enjoy life live longer, they're less accident-prone, and they are less likely to succumb to illness. Enjoying life is in itself a worthy goal: pleasure is a good thing. The place of ecstasy we can reach through sex is also a powerful creative energy that can carry us beyond the limits of the physical world.

Judy Grahn writes specifically about lesbian sex, but her concepts are of equal value to heterosexuals. In her book, *Another Mother Tongue* (Beacon Press, 1990), she describes four sexual "domains," that is, four areas of sexual awareness. The first is the physical: having a good, enjoyable, functional experience. The second is the mental: using fantasy, mental control, and the power of the mind. The third is the psychic: experiencing another realm of existence, beyond intellectual images. The fourth she calls the transformational domain, and she describes it as:

The powers released in this dimension can influence not only the participants but also the world around them and its future.

In my own experience, the energy that gathers and releases when we are sexual is very powerful. It has enormous potential for healing and transformation.

So having a good time is not the only thing to consider when you are having sex. The energy we bring to sex is inseparable from the energy we bring to life, and the healing power of sex affects our lives on a much deeper level than we may realize. By learning how to use this energy consciously, we can change our lives, or dare I say it, change the world. Obviously such a powerful tool needs to be used responsibly. When I try to define responsible sex, I find I cannot separate it from leading a responsible life.

Responsible Sex, Responsible Living

Acting responsibly means acting with compassion. Being
compassionate means being respectful of all beings, including ourselves. It is this last piece that we tend to miss out on.
Too few of us grow up with a sense of our own self-worth
and our right to self-determination. We don't live in a society
that lovingly encourages us to live up to our full potential.
Most of us grow up unaware that there are many different
choices to be made, many different paths to follow. Many of
us are deeply wounded and don't even know it until we accidentally stumble upon a path of healing.

Yes, we need to be loved. We also need to love ourselves.
We need to develop a sense of our own self-worth: worth
that has nothing to do with our accomplishments in the
world, and everything to do with who we are. A sense of self-
worth allows us to tap into our inner power. We can hinder
each other from experiencing self-worth by putting each
other down. Respect is an integral component of
compassion, and compassion is nonjudgmental love. When
we experience nonjudgmental love from another being, it
enables us to accept ourselves, and this in turn allows us to
experience our own inner power. When we experience inner
power, we no longer feel a need to exert power over others,
to force others to agree with us, to prove that we know the
answers and everyone else is wrong. Inner power is nonjudgmental, and respects other people's choices.

Love that disempowers is not true love, and power that
does not come from inside, that does not respect other peo-

ple, is not true power. **True power is always loving and true loving is always empowering**. Loving one another, and especially children, is vital, but if it isn't coupled with the right to self-determination, it is useless. We must teach our children respect, and we can only do this by offering it to them; that means allowing them to make their own decisions about what is right and wrong for them.

Self-esteem, self-respect, and self-worth are all the same thing, and when they are present in an individual, that person is automatically self-empowered.

Working with Energy

Responsible living involves being able to channel our energy so it doesn't harm other people. A feeling is energy, whether it is physical, sexual, intuitive, or emotional. We can choose what to do with the energy that grows out of feelings. For instance, if we feel angry, we can channel it into chopping wood; we can yell at the kids; we can channel it into an orgasm; we can kick the dog; we can rant.

Sometimes the rant is not about whatever is actually making us angry; we can rant on anything we choose. The reason for ranting is the same as the reason for kicking the dog: we are feeling a need to express the energy of the anger. Sometimes we substitute a more acceptable target for our anger, since we are told that we ought to have a good reason for being angry, but this is dishonest. We usually indulge in this dishonesty to protect ourselves: because it is too painful, or it feels futile, to think about the real reasons for our anger, or because we are ashamed of those reasons. I am not saying no one should be angry; there are many good reasons to be angry, and many things to be angry about. But responsible living includes the integrity to acknowledge the real reasons for our anger, instead of fixating on a convenient outlet and blaming others.

Sometimes the original energy was not the energy of anger, but expressing it as anger makes us feel safer, less vulnerable than the original feeling. This is why so many women get impatient with men when men start to express their feelings: because the first feeling that comes up for a man who has been trained to be tough and "manly" is nearly always anger. Anger often covers over other feelings and it isn't always easy to wait for a man to wade through his anger before he gets to what we see as the "real" feelings.

Responsible living involves taking responsibility for what we do with the energy of our feelings, and if necessary, following that energy back to its source in order to prevent it from harming others. It means choosing not to kick the dog (kicking the dog can take many forms, from racial hatred to sexism to child abuse). It means listening to and honoring yourself. It means acknowledging your feelings and needs. And this requires absolute integrity.

Energy is what keeps us alive. That's why we often feel good after we have allowed a strong feeling to flow through us, when we've just had a good rant, or chopped a lot of wood, or had a great orgasm. We feel more alive. We feel energized. All energy is basically life-force energy. When this life-force energy is heightened, speeded up, intensified, life becomes brighter. We are always looking for that which brightens and enriches; that search is part of being alive. We find it in sex and in the expression of feelings, but we also find it in politics, in music, in sports, in art, in raising a family, in a casual exchange with a friendly person on the street, in watching a good movie, in planting a garden and watching it grow, in the deeply rewarding intimacy with someone we have known and loved a long time, in a delighted child's laughter, in a glorious sunset, in ocean waves smashing on rocks. Whenever we are deeply moved by something, whenever we really believe in something, whenever we feel passionate about something, we experience a sense of rightness, which is very exciting.

The energy of the excitement that we are tapping into in any of these situations is the same energy as sexual excitement. Like sex, we can experience this excitement alone: looking at a beautiful view, climbing a mountain, hang-gliding. Or we can experience it with others: when a group of people feel it together the energy is amplified; there is a group euphoria that results in a special kind of bonding. The sense of unity that we experience when we participate in a political rally, sing in a choir, or play team sports is the same unity that we experience when we are in love and having great sex. The problem is that it usually happens so unconsciously that we fixate on whatever happens to bring up the feeling. One person might experience it having sex, and another might experience it at a political rally.

There is a sexual high from singing in choir, for instance; erotic is not quite the right word but it's something like that. I used to feel it much more in rehearsals. Having the audience there was a distraction. Singing in rehearsals was breathtaking. — Joani Blank

People who are not already empowered don't realize that they can make conscious choices about where and when to feel this energy. If they stumble upon it unexpectedly, get caught up in the hysteria of the moment, and unthinkingly attempt to recreate whatever it was that first gave them that wonderful feeling, what may result are religious zealots, sports fanatics, bigots, and "patriots." Find something that looks like it might be a good cause, find someone with a charismatic presence, and you will find people marching in unison, cheering and stomping their feet. They are experiencing their collective energy as very powerful, and it may be the only time in their lives that they feel such a sense of power. It gives them a rush. They feel energized and alive. They have found a way of tapping into the energy of life.

Like a woman who falls in love with someone with whom she experiences a great sexual rush, disempowered people fall in love with whatever it is that creates that rush, and like a woman in love, they want to make it last forever. They lose the ability to discriminate between good sense and manipulative lies. They fail to understand that the ecstasy comes from within themselves. But worst of all, they often get caught up in a kind of mass hysteria that can quickly become violent. Developing the ability to tap into conscious empowerment enables us to make choices: to channel that energy into love and creativity instead of violence and destruction.

Empowerment

We've got to help people understand that the level of ecstasy and passion they undoubtedly feel when they are standing in crowds being carried by a crazy orator is not so different from the transcendental experience we have in our very best sexual encounter. — Joani Blank

An individual who is aware of her (or his) personal power does not lose herself in an energy rush. She does not lose herself at all. Power is simply another word for energy. She knows she can recreate that sense of quickening energy whenever she wants, because she experiences herself as powerful, she is aware of the flow of power within herself. A person who is aware of her inner power is aware of the life-force energy that comes from inside, and this internal energy works in conjunction with external energy.

The alignment of the internal with the external occurs when you acknowledge the forces that motivate you and consciously work with them rather than against them. This is what I call integrity. When you consciously choose a path of integrity, the opportunities that present themselves are exactly right for you. Your energy will be in synchronicity with the energy of the universe. Feelings, attractions, desires, and needs arise from good sense and inner wisdom, and they lead you wherever you need to be. The direction of your life may not be clear until you have gone a little way down the path, and then you will see that it is exactly right. When you arrive at this place, you will fall in love at the right times with the right people. But if you aren't there yet, and if you are not on a path of change and growth, then your feelings, attractions, desires, and needs may be toxic to you. If you are at odds with yourself, then you will be at odds with the energy of the universe.

We can choose to accept the stereotypical ways of being in the world, and live in fear of being abnormal, or we can choose instead to take an active role in challenging those stereotypes within ourselves and outside ourselves. In my opinion, the latter course is the one that offers us the broader future. It is my hope that it is the path you will choose.

Resources

Sex Education and Information

SIECUS
Sexuality Information and Education Council of the United States
130 W. 42nd St., Suite 350, New York, NY 10036-7802
(212) 819-9770
http://www.siecus.org

Coalition for Positive Sexuality
3712 North Broadway, #191 Chicago, IL 60613
(312) 604-1654
http://www.positive.org

San Francisco Sex Information
PO Box 881254, San Francisco, CA 94118
(415) 989-7374
http://www.sfsi.org

The STD Homepage
http://med-www.bu.edu/people/sycamore/std/std.htm
sycamore@bu.edu

Sexual Health Infocenter
http://www.sexhealth.org/infocenter
support@sexhealth.org

The Safer Sex Page
http://www.safersex.org
ss-admin@safersex.org

Planned Parenthood
http://www.plannedparenthood.org
communications@ppfa.org

Society for Human Sexuality
http://www.sexuality.org
humsex@u.washington.edu

Videos, Toys, Books, and Supplies

Blowfish
2261 Market St., #284, San Francisco, CA 94114
(800) 325-2569 or 415 252-4340
http://www.blowfish.com.
Catalog only

Eve's Garden
119 W. 57th St., #420, New York, NY 10019-2383
(800) 848-3837 or (212) 757-8651
Retail store and catalog of toys, books, and videos

Good Vibrations
1210 Valencia St., San Francisco, CA 94110
(415) 974-8990
____
2504 San Pablo Ave., Berkeley, CA 94702
(800) 289-8423
http://www.goodvibes.com
Probably the best source of sex toys, books, and videos for women
of all sexual orientations. Retail stores and mail-order catalog.
Excellent educational and recreational videos with a rating system.
The staff is mostly women who are trained to be both discreet
and helpful.

Toys in Babeland
711 E. Pike St., Seattle, WA 98122
(800) 658-9119 or (206) 658-9119
Retail store and catalog of toys, books, and videos

Xandria Collection
165 Valley Dr., Brisbane, CA 94005
(800) 242-2823 or (415) 463-3812
Mail-order catalog of toys, books, and videos

Organizations

Human Awareness Institute
1730 S. Amphlett Blvd, Suite 225, San Mateo, CA 94402
(800) 800-4117
Workshops on love, intimacy and sexuality

Skydancing Institute
28 Laurel Avenue, San Anselmo, CA 94960
(415) 456-7310
Workshops on Tantra

Body Electric School
6527-A Telegraph Ave., Oakland, CA 94609
(510) 653-1594
Workshops on erotic spirituality

Recommended Reading

What other people do:

Good Sex: Real Stories from Real People, Julia Hutton. Cleis Press.

Shared Intimacies, Lonnie Barbach and Linda Levine. Bantam Books.

My Secret Garden: Women's Sexual Fantasies, and *Women On Top,* Nancy Friday. Pocket Books.

I Am My Lover, Joani Blank. Down There Press.

Sex for One: The Joy of Selfloving, Betty Dodson. Crown Trade Paperbacks.

First Person Sexual: Women And Men Write about Self-Pleasuring, Joani Blank. Down There Press.

The Hite Report, Shere Hite. Dell Publishing.

Ultimate Pleasure: The Secrets of Easily Orgasmic Women, Marc and Judith Meshorer. St. Martin's Press.

How to:

The New Good Vibrations Guide to Sex, Cathy Winks and Anne Semans. Cleis Press.

For Yourself: the Fulfillment of Female Sexuality, Lonnie Barbach. New American Library.

Becoming Orgasmic. Julia Heimann and Joseph Lopiccolo, Fireside Books.

A Hand in the Bush: The Fine Art of Vaginal Fisting, Deborah Addington. Greenery Press.

The Art of Sexual Ecstasy, Margo Anand. Tarcher Press (A classic on simplified tantric sex).

The Ultimate Guide to Anal Sex for Women, Tristan Taormino. Cleis Press.

Extended Sexual Orgasm, Alan and Donna Brauer. Warner Books.

Exhibitionism for the Shy: Show Off, Dress Up and Talk Hot, Carol Queen. Down There Press.

The Ethical Slut, Dossie Easton and Catherine A. Liszt. Greenery Press. (An absolute must for anyone who is thinking about non-monogamy, or wants to understand how non-monogamy can work.)

The Great Sex Weekend: A 48-Hour Guide to Rekindling Sparks for Bold, Busy or Bored Lovers, Pepper Schwartz, Ph.D and Janet Lever, Ph.D. Putnam Publishing Group.

Sensuous Magic: A Guide for Adventurous Couples, Pat Califia. Masquerade Books. (If you are interested in investigating dominance and submission or sadomasochism, this book will give you some ideas about how to do so safely.)

General information:

Femalia. Joani Blank, Down There Press (An illustrated reference on female genital anatomy.)

Good Vibrations: The Complete Guide to Vibrators. Joani Blank, Down There Press.

The Good Vibrations Guide: The G-Spot. Cathy Winks. Down There Press.

The G Spot and Other Recent Discoveries about Human Sexuality, Alice Kahn Ladas, Beverley Whipple, and John Perry. Dell Publishing. (A classic, written by academics, but in a very readable style.)

A New View of a Woman's Body, The Federation of Feminist Women's Health Centers, Feminist Health Press, and *The New Our Bodies, Ourselves,* The Boston Women's Health Collective, Touchstone Books.

Women's Bodies, Women's Wisdom, Christiane Northrup. Bantam Books 1994. (A comprehensive guide to women's health.)

The politics of sex:

Are We Having Fun Yet? Douglas and Douglas. Hyperion. (Why women are not getting fulfillment and some ideas on how they can).

Real Live Nude Girl: Chronicles of Sex-Positive Culture, Carol Queen. Cleis Press.

The Beauty Myth: How Images Of Beauty Are Used Against Women. Naomi Wolf. Anchor. (Exposes the ways in which our judgments of beauty are shaped).

Promiscuities: An Ordinary American Childhood, Naomi Wolf. Random House. (Clearly describes how and why girls in America grow up confused).

Relationships

Peer Marriage: How Love Between Equals Really Works, Pepper Schwartz. The Free Press.

Do I Have To Give Up Me To Be Loved By You? Drs. Jordan and Margaret Paul. Compcare Publishers.

After the Honeymoon: How Conflict Can Improve Your Relationship, Daniel B. Wile. John Wiley and Sons.

For Each Other: Sharing Sexual Intimacy, Lonnie Barbach, Ph.D. Signet Books.

Journey of The Heart: The Path of Conscious Love, John Welwood. Harperperennial Library.

Sexual healing

The Courage To Heal, Laura Davis and Ellen Bass. Harperperennial Library. (The classic on healing from childhood sexual abuse.)

The Sexual Healing Journey: A Guide for Survivors of Sexual Abuse, Wendy Maltz. Harper Collins.

The Healing Woman (bimonthly magazine), The Healing Woman Foundation, PO Box 28040, San Jose, CA 95159. Healing@healing-woman.org

The Obsidian Mirror. Louise Wisechild. Seal Press. (A compelling personal story of healing from abuse.)

Energy flows and the chakra system

The Wheels of Life: A User's Guide to the Chakra System, Anodea Judith. Llewellyn Publications.

Eastern Body, Western Mind: Psychology and the Chakra System as a Path to the Self, Anodea Judith. Celestial Arts.

Hands of Light: A Guide to Healing Through the Human Energy Field, Barbara Ann Brennan. Bantam Books.

Anatomy of the Spirit: The Seven Stages of Power and Healing, Caroline Myss. Three Rivers Press

Information for lesbians and gays, and potential lesbians and gays, may be obtained at: Queer Resources Directory
http://www.qrd.org/ staff@qrd.org

Lesbian presses include Firebrand Books, Seal Press, and Naiad Press. There are remarkably few books written for women who are presently living as heterosexuals, but interested in investigating the lesbian world. The following books may help:

The Straight Woman's Guide To Lesbianism, Mikaya Heart. Wildheart Books.

Lesbian Sex, JoAnn Loulan. Spinsters, Ink

The Original Coming Out Stories, Julia Penelope and Susan J. Wolfe (editors). Crossing Press. (Some very moving personal stories of women's first experience of loving other women.)

Boots Of Leather, Slippers Of Gold: The History of a Lesbian Community. Elizabeth Lapovsky Kennedy and Madeline D. Davis. Penguin USA.

Questionnaire

1. What is your age? 18-28 / 29-39 /40-52 / 53-65 / 66-79 / 80 +

2. Do you identify as: lesbian / bisexual / heterosexual / other
   _____

3. Are you: in relationship(s) and sexually active
   in relationship(s) and not sexually active
   not in relationship(s) and sexually active
   not in relationship(s) and not sexually active
   other _____

4. On a scale of one to ten — one being someone who thinks about sex and wants to do it all the time, and ten being someone who is not interested in sex at all — where would you place your-self? very   1   2   3   4   5   6   7   8   9   10   not

5. Do you talk with your friends and/or lover(s) about sex?
   yes / no / sometimes / other _____

6. As a child, were you discouraged from touching your genitals?
   yes / no / don't remember / other _____

7. Do you remember being touched inappropriately as a child?
   yes / no / not sure / other _____

8. If "Yes" to #7 have you done any healing around it?
   no / a little / lots / other _____

9. Do you think your childhood experience with sex has affected your ease or otherwise with having orgasms? yes / no / maybe / N/A / other _____

10. How often do you have sex (apart from masturbation)?
   never / every day / once or twice a week / other _____

If there have been other times in your life when you've had sex a lot more or a lot less, please explain what you think influences the frequency.

11a. Do you masturbate? yes / no / other _____

b. If yes, do you enjoy it? yes / no / N/A / other _____

c. How often do you masturbate? every day / once or twice a week / once or twice a month / once or twice a year / other _____

If there have been other times in your life when you've masturbated a lot more or a lot less, please explain what you think influences the frequency.

d. Do you generally experience orgasm when you masturbate? yes / no / N/A / usually / that's why I masturbate

12. Have you been able to explain to your lover(s) exactly how to pleasure you ? yes / no / I don't know what to tell them / N/A other _____

13. When you have sex with another person do you most often experience fulfillment / frustration / boredom / joy / satisfaction other _____

14a. Do you dream about sex? If so, are they satisfying dreams? yes / no / other _____

b. Do you physically experience orgasm in these dreams? yes / no / other _____

Please write about your dreams in detail.

15a. Have you ever used a vibrator? yes / no / other _____

b. If yes, did/do you enjoy it? yes / no / somewhat / other _____

16a. Do you like having your clitoris stroked by someone's fingers? yes / no / sometimes / usually / I've never experienced it other _____

b. Do you like having your clitoris orally stimulated? yes / no / sometimes / usually / I've never experienced it / other _____

c. Do you come more easily when you are receiving clitoral stimulation? yes / no / maybe / N/A / other _____

d. Can you come from clitoral stimulation alone?   yes / no / sometimes / N/A / other _____

e. How would you describe to someone how to stimulate you orally?

17a. Do you like vaginal penetration? yes / no / sometimes / usually / I've never experienced it / other _____

b. Do you come more easily when being vaginally stimulated?
yes / no / maybe / N/A / other _____

c. Can you come from vaginal penetration alone? yes / no / sometimes / N/A / other _____

d. Are you aware of your G spot? yes / no / sometimes / other ____

e. What does it feel like when you touch it yourself?

f. What does it feel like when someone else touches it?

18a. Do you like anal penetration? yes / no / usually / sometimes / I've never experienced it / other _____

b. Do you come more easily when being anally stimulated?
yes / no / maybe / N/A / other _____

c. Can you come from anal penetration alone? yes / no / sometimes / N/A / other _____

19a. Have you ever had sex with a man? yes / no

b. If yes, have you had orgasms during sex with a man? yes / no / N/A / other _____

c. Did they occur during: vaginal penetration / anal penetration / clitoral stimulation / other _____

d. If you have had intercourse with a man, was your first time enjoyable / unpleasant / boring / other _____

20a. Have you ever had sex with another woman? yes / no

b. If yes, have you had orgasms during sex with a woman? yes / no / N/A / other _____

c. Did they occur during: vaginal penetration / anal penetration / clitoral stimulation / other _____

d. When you're making love with another woman, how important is it to you that she have an orgasm? very / somewhat / not at all / other _____

21a. Female ejaculation occurs in some women, when they flood or squirt a watery fluid that is similar to but different from urine. Do you ejaculate?

b. If yes, can you tell when you are about to ejaculate? yes / no / sometimes / other _____

c. Is your ejaculation associated with an orgasm? yes / no / sometimes / N/A / other _____

d. What does ejaculate smell like to you, and does it vary at different times?

22a. Are there other parts of your body, besides your genitals, that you find erotic? If so, what parts?

b. Can you orgasm just from having that part(s) stimulated?
yes / no / sometimes / N/A / other _____

23a. Do you have sexual fantasies? yes / no / other _____

b. If yes, do you have them when you are: with another person / alone / either?

c. Do they contribute to your orgasms? yes / no / maybe / N/A / other _____

24a. If you are someone who has experienced vaginal penetration, were you aware of your hymen breaking?

b. Did you bleed? yes / no / other _____

c. Was it painful? yes / no / other _____

If you don't have orgasms, or don't know, skip to question 37

25a. Do you have orgasms when you are: being sexual with another person / masturbating / both / fantasizing / other _____

b. Is there a specific activity that always brings you to orgasm when it is done correctly? If yes, please describe that activity.

26a. No two orgasms are exactly alike, however, some women experience distinct, separate types. Some have what they call clitoral or vaginal orgasms. Do you? yes / no / other _____

Please list the types of orgasm you have, clarifying what differentiates each type, and what has to be done to make them occur.

27a. Do you ever have multiple orgasms (several orgasms one after another with very little interval in between)? yes / no / other

_____

b. If you experience more than one type of orgasm, is one more likely to be multiple? yes / no / N/A / other _____

c. If yes, which type? _____

28a. Do you expect to experience orgasm when someone is making love to you? yes / no / only with some lovers / other _____

b. Do you feel disappointed if you don't? yes / no / other _____

c. If you're disappointed, do you show your lover how you feel? yes / no / sometimes / other _____

29. Have you ever had a one-time experience of orgasm that was quite different from anything else you've experienced? If so, please describe it in detail.

30a. Can you remember the first time you experienced orgasm?

b. If yes, how old were you and what was going on?

c. During your teen years, did you experience orgasm: regularly / sometimes / never / other _____

d. Did you ever experience orgasm in your pre-teen years? yes / no / don't remember

31. Can you isolate anything that makes it more likely you would have an orgasm: for instance, when you are very relaxed; when you're feeling emotionally open; when you're with a stranger; when your clitoris is being orally stimulated; when your clitoris is being manually stimulated; with a vibrator; when your partner is clearly very excited; when you are being penetrated; when you have your legs stretched out straight; when you're with someone

who stimulates you intellectually; when your nipples are being touched; when your partner takes control over you; when you take control over your partner; when you're alone. Please write what brings you to orgasm in as much detail as you can, using a separate sheet of paper.

32. Would you describe your orgasms as any of the following: exquisite / deep / clenching / pounding / electrical / like riding a wave / like falling / like flying / like an earthquake / other

_____

Please write in your own words what orgasm, and the buildup to it, are like for you. Be as detailed as you can!

33a. Can you have an orgasm when you are sexually stimulating your lover, but your body is not being stimulated (you're not rubbing on anything and no one is touching you)? yes / no / other

_____

b. If yes, how often has this happened? What do you think allows it to happen?

c. Can you have an orgasm when you are not touching anyone else, and your body is not being sexually stimulated (that is, nobody is touching you, and you are not touching yourself or rubbing on anything)? yes / no / other _____

d. If yes, how often has this happened and what were the circumstances?

34. After having an orgasm, or orgasms, are you energized / sleepy / other _____

35. Have you ever faked orgasm? yes / no / other _____

If yes, under what circumstances, and why?

36. Do you have more powerful orgasms when you make a lot of noise? yes / no / don't know / other _____

For women who don't have orgasms: Please write what it is you like, or liked, about any of the stimulation described in the previous questions.

37. Do you ever feel like you're close to having an orgasm but can't quite get there? yes / no / often / other _____

38. Do you have clearly identifiable peaks in your sexual enjoyment? yes / no / sometimes / other _____

39a. Why do you think you don't have orgasms?

40a. Do you tell other people that you don't have orgasms? yes / no / other _____

b. If yes, what kind of reactions do you get when you tell other people? If no, what kind of reactions do you think you would get?

c. How do/would those reactions make you feel?

d. What kind of reaction would you like to get?

40a. Do you feel deprived or frustrated because you don't have an experience you can clearly label orgasm? yes / no / other _____

b. Do you wish you had a clearly identifiable orgasmic response? yes / no / other _____

c. Have you done anything specifically to try and have orgasms? yes / no / other _____

d. If yes, what?

e. Have you attended or considered attending a workshop on how to have orgasms? yes / no / maybe / other _____

f. Do you have a clear idea of something that you feel would be helpful to you in learning to experience orgasms? If so, what?

Index

RAISING A DAUGHTER
Parents and the Awakening of a Healthy Woman
by Jeanne and Don Elium

This dynamic husband and wife team bring their special expertise to the unique and often daunting challenges of nurturing little girls into confident young women. Covering the stages from infancy, through the teen years, and on into young adulthood, *Raising A Daughter* is not only indispensible reading for parents, but because every woman is a daughter, it also offers illuminating insight on what it means to be female.

ISBN 0-89087-708-4
available in hardcover or quality paperback

GIRLS TO WOMEN, WOMEN TO GIRLS
by Bunny McCune and Deb Traunstein

At a time when hormones, peer pressure, and messages from the media can profoundly affect the choices our teenagers make, *Girls to Women* offers some voices of sanity as females of all ages share the experience of transitioning into womanhood. Topics include: maintaining a healthy body image; "fitting in" without losing a sense of self; understanding the mother/daughter relationship; and first sexual experiences. *Girls to Women* will appeal to preteens and up.

ISBN 0-89087-881-1
available in quality paperback

THE WOMAN'S GUIDE TO PEAK PERFORMANCE
by Susan Puretz, Adelaide Haas, and Donna Meltzer, M.D.

Packed with information and encouragement, this is the ultimate fitness primer geared especially to women of all ages and at all levels of health.

ISBN 0-89087-841-2
available in quality paperback

EASTERN BODY, WESTERN MIND
Psychology and the Chakra System as a Path to the Self
by Anodea Judith

Modern psychology meets and mingles with the ancient Hindu chakra system of subtle energy to create a unique synthesis of Eastern tradition and Western science.

ISBN 0-89087-815-3
available in quality paperback

STUMBLING TOWARD ENLIGHTENMENT
by Geri Larkin

Having evolved (by popular demand) from the dharma talks given by the author at the Ann Arbor Buddhist Temple and the Chicago Zen Buddhist Temple, her style is honest and earthy and even a little scrappy. This is accessible Zen from the heartland with humorous twists from a woman's perspective.

ISBN 0-89087-849-8
available in quality paperback

LOVING SOMEONE GAY
revised & updated 3rd edition
by Don Clark, Ph.D.

For three decades, Dr. Don Clark has offered courageous and compassionate guidance to gay men and women, their friends, families and loved ones, and the professionals who work with them.

ISBN 0-89087-705-X
available in quality paperback

JOURNAL TO INTIMACY
A Couple's Journal for Sustaining Love
by Rose Offner

Whether you are beginning a new relationship, healing an old one, or maintaining a current one—the key to every relationship is self-exploration through self-revelation. Color, imagery, and visual metaphors speak to the soul in this interactive journal for couples to share.

ISBN 0-89087-873-0
available in quality paperback

For more information on Celestial Arts titles, you may write to us at:

P.O. Box 7123 Berkeley, CA 94707

or visit us on our web site: www.tenspeed.com

to order by phone: (800)841-BOOK

or by e-mail: order@tenspeed.com